Doing it with Pete

The Lighten Up Slimming Fun Book

Pete Cohen & Judith Verity

Foreword *by* **Roger Black** MBE

Crown House Publishing, Bancyfelin, Carmarthen, Wales

Published in the UK by

Crown House Publishing Ltd
Crown Buildings
Bancyfelin
Carmarthen
Wales

First published 1999

British Library of Cataloguing-in-Publication Data
A catalogue entry for this book is available
from the British Library.

ISBN 1899836195

Printed and bound in Wales by
WBC Book Manufacturers,
Waterton Industrial Estate,
Bridgend, Mid Glamorgan.

*The characters in this book are fictional. Any resemblance to any individual,
whether living or dead, is purely coincidental.*

Dedication

I would like to dedicate this book to all the people I have worked with over the last thirteen years. You taught me so much. To all of you who let me share the changes you made in your lives. I couldn't have written this book without you.

Thank you.

~Peter Cohen

About the Authors

Pete Cohen

Pete Cohen has worked in the Health and Fitness industry for twelve years as a sports psychologist, personal trainer and lecturer in sports science and nutrition, and he is well known for his work with teams and individuals. He is currently working as sports psychologist and motivator to Kent County Cricket club and the British Blind Cricket Team as well as with a number of well-known athletes.

Seven years ago, Pete developed the Lighten Up weight control method using sports psychology techniques, NLP, and much of his own insight and wisdom. Lighten Up has proved hugely successful and his audiotape and first book, *Slimming With Pete*, have become hugely popular.

Unlike many other slimming gurus, Pete doesn't have a weight problem himself. But, if you ask him whether he really understands the desperation of people caught in the dieting trap, he will tell you he has plenty of experience in overcoming problems and succeeding in the face of enormous difficulties. Diagnosed severely dyslexic as a child and told that further education would be out of the question, he now has more degrees than GCSEs as well as a best-selling book to his name. Pete Cohen is one of those people who never gives up on a problem until he finds the solution.

His warmth, energy and enthusiasm have made him hugely popular on TV and in the media, but he is a natural entertainer and teacher and, for him, there is no substitute for working directly with the people he is helping. So, his work as a sports psychologist continues and he still runs his inspirational Lighten Up workshops and eight-week evening courses. Although he isn't able to do as many of these as he would like, there is a weekend workshop every month and a new evening course every ten weeks.

Working with Pete is always a memorable and life-enhancing experience.

Judith Verity

Judith Verity has twenty-eight years of varied experience as a probation officer, counsellor, trainer, businesswoman and writer. In the 1980s she ran her own training and office management company, eventually selling out in order to concentrate on teaching and writing. She has a particular interest in dieting problems and has worked with people suffering from eating disorders. When she met Pete Cohen and he told her his story, she was so inspired by it that they decided to work together to put Lighten Up into writing. This is their second book, the first being *Slimming With Pete* which was the story of Pete's first group.

Table of Contents

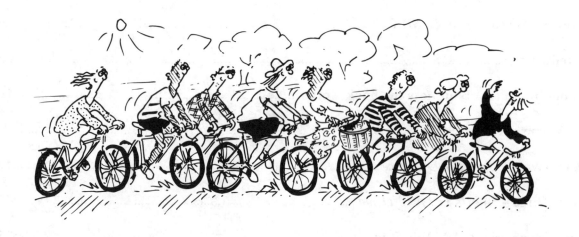

Acknowledgments

My Mum and Dad, for just being who you are – the best parents in the world.

Colin and Shellie Deans, for your work on the programme and especially to Colin for giving me my first break all those years ago.

Helena Boycott, thank you for being so helpful and creative, for letting us use your picture and for your recipes.

David Schweitzer, for your support and help. Love and light.

Paul McKenna and Michael Breen, for your support and for the training that has inspired and motivated me.

Richard Bandler, the originator of NLP and other contributors in this field, some of whose techniques and ideas have been used in this book.

Special thanks to Gretchen Mackay, Mitch and Tina Powis, and Richard and Valerie Curen.

Roger Black, for your kind words and support.

Grizelda, thank you for the great illustrations.

John, who takes final responsibility for all the glitches, typos and inconsistencies that he missed.

Maria, you took the world off our shoulders so that we could meet our deadline.

Andy Sellins, for being my best mate.

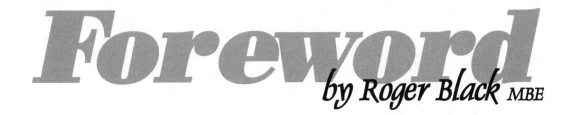
Foreword
by Roger Black MBE

I met Pete Cohen through his work as a sports psychologist, so I was surprised to hear that he'd written a book about slimming. Now that I've read it, I can see the connection. Pete has put into this book all the expertise and commitment that has made him a successful coach and motivator to so many top athletes.

It's fun to read and full of sound, solid, good advice with techniques that really work. Pete and I both believe that the key to success is to have inspiring, compelling personal goals and put your heart into reaching them. Pete takes it a step further and shows you how to achieve your dream of becoming fitter and slimmer for the rest of your life.

In the competitive world of athletics there are a lot of people who want to be champions, but, sadly, there's only room at the top for a few. Slimming isn't like that – everyone can be a winner – although it seems to me that slimming and athletics do have something in common. Why is it that some athletes and some slimmers achieve their goals, while others never quite make it? The answer is so obvious it's easy to miss: the second-rate athletes and the permanently overweight dieters are using the wrong approach. They both spend too much time focusing on what they don't want and doubting whether they will succeed. Pete's message for dieters is the same as his training for athletes: 'Focus on what you want and dump the doubts.'

Slimmers, like athletes, need to exercise. The problem is that most people think exercise has to be hard and painful. Well, to be honest, if you want to run 400 metres competitively, then your training is likely to be tough. But if your goal is to be slim, it doesn't have to be so intense. Sure, you need to exercise, but gently. And you need to make changes to your diet as well, but, as Pete points out, that's about eating the right things, not about constantly fretting over what you aren't allowed.

The techniques Pete uses with top athletes and sportspeople as well as with many people who have already become permanently slimmer is now available to you. He can move you (literally) to become permanently slimmer, fitter and healthier.

Whether you want to be an Olympic medallist or whether you want to just lose weight, you go about it the same way: first, get the right information and second, learn how to focus on your desired outcome with passion and determination.

I've seen Pete make a difference to people's lives and I believe that this book will make a difference to yours. If you follow the Lighten Up programme you will learn how to get pleasure from being more active and eating a healthier, more balanced diet. And I can tell you that it's a lifestyle you'll want to keep once you've got it.

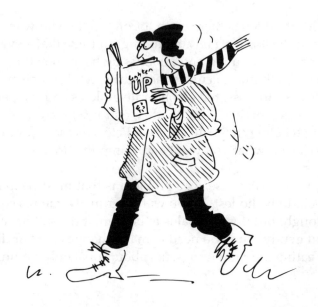

Introduction

Seven years ago, Pete noticed that many of his clients had a hidden agenda – they were more concerned with weight loss than fitness. He decided to work directly with this problem and set out to do his own research into weight control and dieting. When he discovered that dieting was part of the problem rather than the solution, he began to develop the Lighten Up method. He was shocked to discover that slimming was an obsession for so many people who spent their lives thinking about food and what they weren't allowed to eat. They'd stopped being themselves and enjoying life. And despite all this suffering, or, as Pete believes, because of it, only 5% of dieters ever manage to maintain their target weight.

Feeding the obsession

Dieting is obsessional behaviour. It's not normal behaviour. And most conventional diets cleverly encourage the obsession – prompting slimmers to count calories, think about what they can't eat and combine food in complicated ways. Focusing on the problem like this feeds the obsession as well as the fat cells.

But we can't blame big business and the media for everything, and ultimately, our own surplus fat is our own responsibility. The first step to staying slim is to acknowledge that. Then we can change. Before Pete wrote this book he studied slim people and people with weight problems and the Lighten Up method is about the difference that makes the difference. The techniques you will read about and put into practice in this book have always been used by slim, healthy people. And by people who used to be overweight until they made positive, permanent changes in their lives.

There are no external solutions (like diets) to an internal problem. Pete is aiming to help you re-learn the knowledge your body was born with. Knowledge which your conscious mind has decided, for lots of social and emotional reasons, to override. This is hardly surprising: there's a lot of social pressure to disconnect yourself from your body's natural regulating system.

When you were a baby you ate only when you were hungry. Your stomach told your brain when it was full. But gradually, you may have been persuaded to eat for other reasons. Parents sometimes feed babies because they don't know why they are crying, and throughout your childhood you were told to finish what was on your plate or to eat because it was breakfast time, regardless of whether you were hungry. You learned that certain foods are treats or rewards and you learned to use food for comfort.

It's no wonder that food holds a vice-like grip on our emotions and that our relationship with it is complex. And often the food we eat in non-hunger situations is sweet and fattening and leaves us feeling miserable and bloated. Whatever we eat when we aren't hungry gets turned into fat and stored for later.

This book is designed to support you in making powerful changes over the next eight weeks as you start to gain more control of your life.

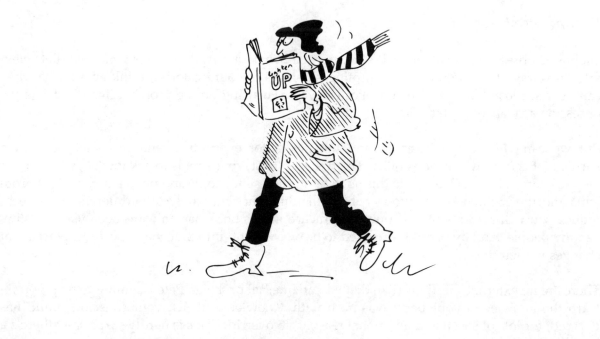

A note from Pete
about how the book works

I designed this book as a step-by-step programme with exercises on the left and information on the right. If you want to make the most effective changes, take your time and read it over the next eight weeks – or however long seems comfortable to you.

There's a lot of information here, so be patient as you focus on the exercises and the questions. At the end of each chapter you will find guidelines for a **Food Diary** as well as a set of **Challenges** for the following week. There's a lot to do, so you won't have time for calorie counting and daily weighing sessions.

Do this first

Buy yourself a notebook or journal and write down your commitment to the programme in the front of it. This will give you a structure and a physical reminder of your motivation. Don't start the exercises until you've done this, because writing good ideas down on random bits of paper (or trying to store them in your head) is hopeless. They'll get lost, and these are changes you want to hang on to.

Exercises

The exercises on the left hand side of the pages are mostly mind games, though I do encourage you to make some new physical moves too.

There are a lot of question and answer sessions. I want you to get them out of your head and down in black and white. Before you let your mind run with insights that will change your life, write down the answers. Writing down an answer fixes the thought and imprints it in your brain. You'll be amazed at just how quickly changes happen once you get into the habit of writing down what you do.

Food Diary and Challenges

I also ask you to keep a **Food Diary** because this will help you to give yourself the support you need as well as providing the most amazing insights into what motivates you and what you need to do in order to change. It's not a new idea, but this is rather more advanced than most because you'll be writing down a lot more than your eating habits.

As you keep your **Diary**, at the end of every chapter, you will be encouraged to widen your attention. Awareness is the first step on the journey of change. A change of mind is the second step towards the shape of things to come.

The **Challenges** are right at the end of each chapter because I want you to take them with you through the week. I hope that, by the time you finish the book, setting **Challenges** for yourself every day will have become a habit for life.

What to do if...

A particular exercise or idea seems be taking a little longer, or you feel that a particular week still needs some attention: just start that week all over again.

You don't see immediate changes: be patient with yourself, as you give yourself time and space to change. This is fairly fundamental stuff we're talking about – there's more to it than adjusting your calorie intake. So wait and see. Be observant and non-judgmental.

If you need more support or advice: write to us or e-mail us at the address at the back of the book. The first book, *Slimming with Pete*, and the audiotape might also give you some useful backup as you travel through the weeks. In fact, the audiotape might be particularly effective because it talks you through some of the exercises.

Let's do it.

Week
A Good Start

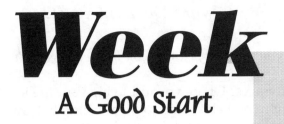

'If you always do what you've always done, you'll always get what you've always got.'

Mo looked up from her cafe latte. 'If you've come here to preach at me, you can go away. If I've heard that quote once I've heard it a thousand times.'

'That quote is a life saver – at least, that's what you told me on New Year's Day,' I reminded her. I decided to sit down anyway. It was the only empty stool I could see – those American coffee shops get very crowded first thing in the morning.

'Yes, I know,' she agreed, 'I had a hangover, remember? Just like I always do, every New Year's Day. But I *don't* have hangovers very often during the rest of the year. And this precious moment in the morning with my coffee and the newspaper is a treat I give myself. Sometimes I even get around to setting outcomes for the day before it starts.' She waved a notebook at me.

'Fair enough. But how did you get to be so thin and glamorous over the past six months when you're still spending your time in coffee shops?'

'The difference is that now I indulge only every couple of days. And I *really* enjoy it. The other mornings I tend to be working out at the health club, in case you hadn't noticed. I don't stuff myself with coffee and croissants all morning like I used to. But occasionally I come in here for an orgasmic breakfast experience and then get on with my life.'

I went up to the bar and ordered an orange juice. There was a queue but when I got back to where Mo was sitting she was sipping slowly and thoughtfully, her cup still half-full.

'So how did you motivate yourself to make the change?' I asked her.

She smiled. 'I hate to tell you this, but I never even noticed myself eating in the morning until you made us keep a diary. Then once I realised I was nibbling all the time and not really enjoying it, I made an agreement with myself not to eat breakfast at work. Either I get some fruit after I've worked out or I treat myself and come here. And this is a great idea because I can't afford to eat too much at these prices!'

'So, you're eternally grateful to me?' I said, hopefully. She gave me a look.

What Do You Expect?

If you always do what you've always done, you'll always get what you've always got...

Have you been dieting for ages? Or are you just living your life in a body that doesn't suit you? However things are, you're probably used to them being that way. Maybe you sometimes get close to the weight you want to be, but do you ever really believe it will last?

But now you've bought, or borrowed, this book. I'll be surprised if it's the first diet book you've bought, but if it is, then all I can say is *First Time Lucky*.

If it's not your first time, I want to ask you to think carefully about what you really want and what you expect to get. This isn't about counting calories, or food combining, or eating before five o'clock. That's just rules, and rules are a piece of cake. Which, as you've often been told, makes you fat.

If you want to go ahead and Lighten Up, make your decision to change right now. The introduction's over and the process starts with the next paragraph.

Over the next eight weeks, or however long you want to take, you'll get used to answering or ignoring the questions I keep asking you. When you look at them, you'll be surprised at how you start thinking about the answers. And how much valuable information you will discover about yourself.

If you've ever tried to lose weight before, what methods have you tried?

Include any plan or behaviour pattern other than eating when you were hungry. From food fads to eating disorders and all the pain and grief in between. Exercise routines which weren't fun should be included too.

What did those methods do for you at the time?

Did you lose any weight? For how long? Did you feel good at the time?

What long-term effects have those diets had on you?

Are you still following any of those routines? Do some of them still haunt you like unhappy ghosts? Did they permanently change your way of life – or your shape – for better or worse?

You already know that diets don't work and you are now starting a new programme. Not one of pain, starvation, denial and confusion. A new programme of self-discovery.

You will learn more about yourself as you start thinking differently and become more aware of exactly what you need to do.

Dieting – A Recipe For Failure

It probably won't surprise you when I tell you that 95% of people who go on a diet put the weight back on again when it's finished. And even with this incredibly low success rate, the diet industry in this country is worth over £1 billion each year. And in the US it's worth $32 billion, making it the fourth largest retail business, in spite of the rapidly rising obesity rate. It's estimated that by 2030, most Americans will be obese, and so will 37% of Brits. And because overweight people are generally less healthy, these statistics imply a really frightening increase in illness and disease.

So let me ask you again, what has dieting done for you? Has it made you slimmer? Has it made you healthier? Has it made you more obsessed with food? Do you know how many calories there are in just about everything? Do you think about food a lot? Are you worried about the fat content of each mouthful you take?

People who diet regularly tend to be obsessed with their weight and they seem to weigh themselves all the time. Some diets encourage people to deny themselves food for long periods so that eventually they binge or overeat. And a lot of them are confusing and complicated.

From all the evidence I've ever seen or heard – and believe me, I've met hundreds of slimmers – most diets are a complete waste of time and money. Worse still, they can actually be dangerous. Eating disorders are on the increase and I sometimes wonder if, in the western world, we are moving towards a situation where most of the population is overweight while the rest are dangerously malnourished. In the late 1980s the average weight of contestants in the Miss America contests was less than the US standard for anorexia. Yet, animals don't diet. It's not normal behaviour. And there are no fat cats or catwalk models in the wild.

So why does the diet business continue to grow and flourish? Well, there are two reasons:

One reason is that the industry keeps coming up with new products, claiming that each new diet is the revolutionary one that will change your life and make you slimmer and healthier for ever. Have you ever heard any of these? *'Lose ten pounds in a week'*, *'Look slimmer in four hours'*, *'Drink yourself thin'*.

The second reason is that it creates its own demand. You start dieting because you want to lose a little weight but, once you've started, it's hard to stop. Once you start counting calories, weighing yourself and worrying all the time about what you can't eat, it's hard to go back to the natural way of eating when you're hungry. Diets deliberately set out to make you dependent on them and often they do it by confusing you about whether you really feel hungry or not.

Did you know, it's estimated now that there are over 330,000 diets in the world? Isn't that crazy when you think about how few people actually get any slimmer?

Health Warning –

Dieting Can Make You Fat

When you look in the **mirror,**

you are looking at the **problem.**

But **remember,**

you are also looking at the *solution.*

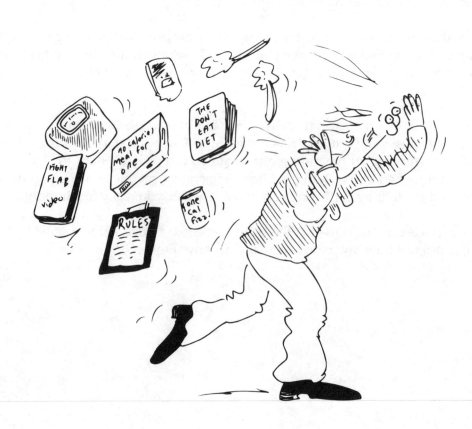

Stop Dieting And Start Living

In the 1940s the University of Minnesota conducted research on the effects of starvation.

A group of normal, psychologically healthy men of normal weight were put on a diet that, like some of today's diet plans, cut their daily calorie intake in half.

The men were closely monitored and over a six-month period their average body weight dropped by twenty-five pounds. The average rate at which their bodies digested food dropped by 40% because their bodies believed they were experiencing famine.

When the diet finished, it took, on average, fourteen months for the men's weight and metabolism to return to normal. And, during that period, every single one of them displayed anorexic, bulimic or binge-eating behaviour patterns.

They had distorted their bodies' natural weight regulation mechanisms and their systems were out of control. To start with, they regained the lost weight plus about 10% extra. And the first weight they put back on was in the form of fat.

Eventually, their weight normalised and their body fat percentages dropped back to their pre-diet levels. But they were being watched and regulated and they knew they were part of an experiment. Most dieters today would panic if they gained back the weight they'd lost plus an extra 10%. In fact, most dieters today do panic, because that's exactly what happens to most of them when they stop dieting. And, when people are alarmed, they tend to take drastic action – like starting another diet when the balance of their metabolism is still disturbed from the last one.

Get off the dieting bandwagon and make friends with your body again. Start listening to it and learn to eat only when you are hungry. Focus on what you want to be: slimmer, fitter and healthier.

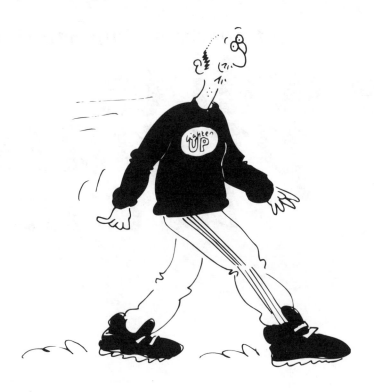

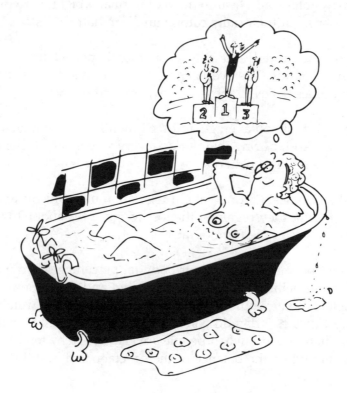

The will to win
is *not* nearly *as important as*
the will to
prepare
to win.

Weight Loss Or Fat Loss?

I often ask people who want to be slimmer what it is that they want and they say things like:

- *'I want to lose weight.'*

- *'I've got to get rid of this fat.'*

- *'I'm determined to shed at least two stone.'*

- *'I'm fed up with looking like the Michelin Man.'*

- *'I hate the way I get out of breath just walking up stairs.'*

This doesn't tell me what they want; it tells me what they don't want, which is excess weight.

Just losing weight is too easy.

If I offered you ten pounds for £4.99, you'd probably say *'ten pounds of what?'* So why do we never ask ourselves that question when we're dieting?

If you drastically cut back on food you will certainly lose weight, but, unfortunately, not much of it will be fat. Our bodies try to protect us. When rations are cut, our bodies assume we are under siege and starving to death. So they promptly slow down the rate at which we digest food and hold on to the source that lasts the longest, which of course is FAT.

Our bodies will even use muscle for energy. So the scales will show real weight loss – but it's not fat loss. Muscle tissue weighs three times as much as fat. What's even worse is that when we stop dieting and go back to our old eating patterns, the weight we lost as muscle comes back on as FAT.

Did you know that it's almost physiologically impossible to lose more than two pounds of fat in a week? Even if you didn't eat a thing for the whole seven days, you might lose a lot of weight but only a couple of pounds of it would be fat. It's a survival mechanism we inherited from our hunting forefathers who didn't know where the next meal was coming from. If you really want to get rid of fat, you have to be patient. Let your body adapt itself comfortably to losing half a pound to two pounds of fat each week. *And don't keep checking.*

The only way to be permanently slimmer is to know what you want and work with your body, not against it.

What Do You Want?

What Do You Want?

Write down the first weight-loss goal that comes into your head. Don't think too deeply about this question. What do you imagine when you write down the answer?

What Do You Want?

You may not need a second attempt at this question if you made a nice, positive statement the first time. But if your answer contains something like:

> **'I mustn't keep eating.'**
>
> **'I want to cut out fat and sugar.'**
>
> **'I don't want to be a size 16 any more.'**

you may find your mind filling up with images of constant eating, slabs of fat, bags of sugar and rails and rails of frumpy size 16s.

Write down something more inspiring next time around. Something that fills your mind with pictures of you looking slim, healthy, happy, glowing and vital.

For example:

> **'I want to be fitter, slimmer and healthier.'**
>
> **'I want to look great in a swimsuit.'**
>
> **'I want to buy fashionable clothes.'**
>
> **'I want to get admiring glances when I walk into a room.'**
>
> **'I want to feel good about myself.'**

Are you ready to write something positive? Something to aim for rather than something you might want to move away from?

Now, with this idea in mind, what do you see? Bring the picture closer and make it brighter, bolder and more real.

Don't Think Of A Pink Elephant

We have a tendency to focus on what's *not* working, that is, on problems. Which is a pity really because our brains work much more efficiently with positive commands. In fact, the human brain deletes negatives.

What happens if I tell you not to think of a **Pink Elephant**? Your brain has to produce one first and then erase it. If you say to yourself, '*I must not keep eating*,' guess what message you get?

Say to yourself, 'I must lose *weight*.' Write down what you see when you say it.

What happens when you say to yourself, 'I am going to *be slimmer*?' What do you picture in your mind?

You get what you focus on. So what exactly have you been focusing on?

Your brain is like a heat-seeking missile. It will home in on whatever is put in front of it. So, tell yourself what you want, *not* what you don't want. If you are watching your weight, that is exactly what you will keep seeing. Depressing, isn't it?

Start putting your aims and goals and dreams for a slimmer future into positive terms. Imagine how an architect has to draw up detailed plans before starting to build a house. Or how a hairdresser is able to picture in his/her mind the very style that's going to make you look good. Your vision of how *you* want to be needs to be as detailed as the architect's drawings. Try writing or drawing a clear description of the new you in your notebook. Then you can refer to it whenever the memory grows dim or you need a flash of inspiration.

As you look at what you've jotted down, a picture may appear in your mind. Perhaps it's already sharply defined, in bright, clear colours. Or maybe it's slowly taking shape. Give it the attention it deserves.

In life you get what you focus on. All great achievers owe their success to their ability to focus exactly on what it is that they want. Haven't you met people like that? They're usually banging on about having a dream or a vision when everybody else is complaining about working long hours for low pay.

Every great achievement flashes through the mind before it turns into reality – or before reality turns into an amazing result.

What Do You Really Want?

DECIDE what you want.
Decide
what you are **willing** *to* exchange for it.

~H L Hunt, *Oil Executive*

Think of something positive that you've done in your life. Something that meant cutting yourself off from other possibilities. Something you made a decision to do and then went ahead and did. And even though there might have been some setbacks, you carried on because you knew, deep down, that you were going to achieve your goal.

It doesn't matter whether it turned out to be right or wrong. It's the process that matters.

- I bought a car.
- I moved to a place of my own.
- I changed jobs.
- I went to college.
- I passed my exams.
- I gave up work to look after the kids.
- I learned to dance.
- I got married.
- I became independent.
- I adopted a cat.
- I started a business.
- I saved up for a holiday.
- I escaped…

Make a firm commitment to be slimmer. Leave yourself no other option.
True commitment to a decision always unlocks the energy to achieve it.

The Power Of Decisions

When you come to a fork in the road, take it!

Yogi Berra.

What precedes all behaviours, actions and performances?

What turns dreams into reality?

The answer is *decisions*. **Your decisions**. They determine what you think, how you feel, what you do and who you become.

Why are some people successful at becoming slimmer, fitter and healthier? Because they make better decisions. Because they make decisions, full stop.

Most of us just hope, wish and, eventually, regret... *'I'm not good enough.' 'I'm too old.' 'I haven't had the right opportunities.' 'I'm just a fat person…'*

Success is no accident. The difference between people who end up slimmer, fitter and healthier and those who don't, has nothing to do with luck (or metabolism). I have noticed consistent, logical, behaviour patterns among successful slimmers.

Successful slimmers take effective action towards getting into shape and everyone can learn from what they do.

This book is about the powerful strategies and techniques for change that I have learned over the years. I can give you the information you need to reach your goal, but there's one ingredient missing and without it, you won't even get past first base. Action is what generates success.

The thought of taking action to become slimmer may be painful. But you are already taking action. It's producing the results you've got now. The results you've got by eating to change the way you feel, by constantly dieting and thinking about food, or by punishing, damaging exercise routines. All of those actions have produced results. Sometimes massive results. But they may not have been the results you wanted.

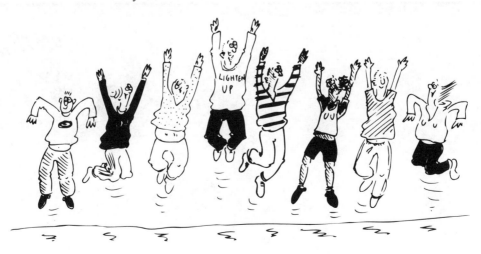

It's *decisions,* *not* conditions, that hold you back.

Contract

- ✸ I'M WILLING TO READ THIS BOOK AND TO HONOUR MY DECISION TO BECOME PERMANENTLY SLIMMER AND HEALTHIER.

- ✸ I WILL WRITE DOWN WHAT I EAT AND DRINK.

- ✸ I WILL USE THE TECHNIQUES AND STRATEGIES IN THIS BOOK AND ADD TO MY LIFE THE ONES THAT WORK OUT FOR ME.

- ✸ I CAN AND WILL SUCCEED.

Signed

Date

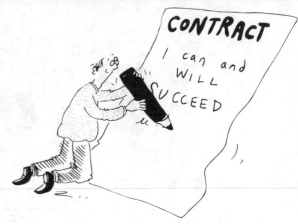

Making A Contract

Watch your thoughts; they become words.

Watch your words; they become actions.

Watch your actions; they become habits.

Watch your habits; they become character.

Watch your character; it becomes your DESTINY.

~ Frank Outlaw

Silly as this may sound, almost every study of success and motivation that's ever been done has found that people who write down their goals are much more likely to achieve them. And the commitment I am suggesting you put your signature to here is a very easy one. All you are agreeing to do is read this book and take on the **Challenges** at the end of each chapter.

The first step I want you to take is to buy yourself a large notebook right away because I'm going to ask you to keep a **Food Diary**.

And, yes, I know there's nothing revolutionary in that. Lots of diet books suggest you do it. Some of them encourage you to write down every calorie you consume. But I don't see the point in that, unless you want to get really obsessional about food and, I suspect, you may have been there and done that already.

And I know there are other diet books that ask you, as I do, to become more aware of your eating patterns. Well, that's because it's very useful to know more about when and where and why and how you eat. What you eat is less important, though I shall be asking you to record that as well – to begin with.

We are all creatures of habit and most of our daily routines are automatic. Writing things down can make you aware of personal patterns you never noticed before. And when you notice a bad habit you can start changing it. If you want to.

You can't tackle a problem you aren't even aware of.

Food Diary 1

Time	Food and Drinks	Activity
6.00am	Small packet Wotsits, Coke	Walking to bus.
10.00am	Bacon sandwich, orange juice	Working.
12.30pm	Kebab and chips, mineral water	Working.
5.00pm	Banana, apple, 2 cups tea	Working.
11.00pm	Curry, rice, 2 pappadoms 2 lagers, 1 coffee	None.

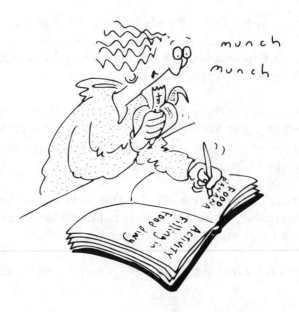

munch
munch

Next Week's Food Diary

For the next eight weeks, I'll be asking you to keep your **Food Diary**. Buy yourself an exercise book and make it a thick one with a strong cover; it's going to be full of useful information that you can refer back to as the weeks go by. At the beginning of each chapter there will be a review of the previous week and it's a good idea to make a few notes in the diary as you answer my questions.

How to be You – The Manual.

Imagine that I have asked you to write me a detailed instruction manual about how to be You for a week. After a few weeks I should have enough detail to copy your eating habits with a high degree of accuracy.

So keep it simple but make sure it's comprehensive. Write down everything at the time you eat it. Don't wait until the end of the day.

At the beginning of the next chapter there's a review of how you got on with this first week's diary. Challenge yourself now to run it for a week at least.

This diary is about you. It may start with what you eat, but it's designed to start you thinking about why you eat and lead on to how you might enjoy it more – and a lot of other things too.

Awareness is the first step on the journey of change. You'll be surprised at what you find out about yourself as you begin now to notice more about what you do and when you do it.

For the first week, make a note of:
- What you eat and drink.
- When you eat and drink.
- Search for patterns in your eating and drinking.
- What are you doing when you're eating?

On the left is an example of someone's **Food Diary.** Not an example I suggest you copy – I put it in just to show you how it might look. Make up your own format; it will vary each week but as long as you include all the information I ask you for, you can lay it out any way you want.

Good luck.

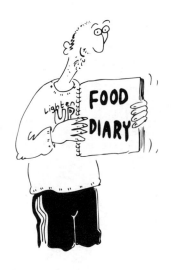

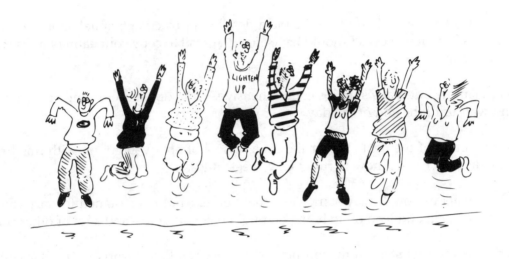

They can because they think they can.

Virgil

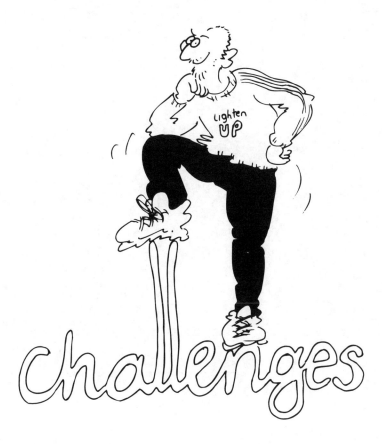

Every week, at the end of the chapter, we will be including some **Challenges** for you. They are to help you get into the habit of regularly challenging yourself to move out of your comfort zone and start to change. For the first week, they are quite simple and straightforward.

➡ **Spend some time each day picturing in your mind what it is that you want, how you will look and how you will feel when you are slimmer, fitter and healthier.**

➡ **Honour your decision to change by telling yourself that you are going to achieve your ideal weight.**

➡ **Write down what you eat and drink.**

➡ **Look to see how active you are on a daily basis.**

➡ **If you are looking for inspiration to cook healthy meals, turn to the back of the book and experiment with some of the recipes. They aren't necessarily meant to be followed to the letter. You can add your own variations to all of them.**

➡ **Look back through this first chapter a couple of times during the week – some things may jump out at you that you missed the first time around.**

➡ **Do all the exercises on the left-hand pages.**

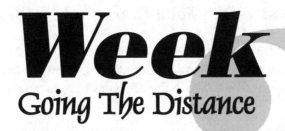

Week
Going The Distance

In a rash moment, over a curry with friends one night, I agreed to help Ben train for a ten kilometre run. I vaguely remember telling him it was all a question of proper training. Next morning he was at my door with the forms. 'Are you sure about this?' I asked him.

'I've made a decision,' he said. 'And now I know I'm going to do it, I want to get started.'

'We'll start right now, if you like. But you're not rushing at it. Pace yourself. It's going to take time.' He knew I meant it, so he agreed. We trained, for four months before the race. The first few weeks were tough; in his rugby days Ben had been fit and ten years younger.

'I don't remember it being this hard', he said, struggling to get his feet into his trainers at six am one morning.

'Try unlacing them first', I suggested.

'No, the training. I used to run first thing in the rugby season and it wasn't this painful. Mind you', he added, 'I didn't do a day's work afterwards, and first thing was ten o'clock.'

But he stuck with it, running through the coldest months. We were eating well and feeling pretty good. One evening he called at the club for his evening workout just as I was going home to watch the match on TV. He looked at me reproachfully. 'I've already done a couple of classes today and a personal training session', I reminded him. 'I do this for a living, remember? My body's had enough and so have I. Why don't you have a night off too?'

'Actually, I've been looking forward to a workout,' he admitted. 'I've been invigilating exams all day and I'm used to being more active now. I'll catch the end of the game with you later.'

On the day of the run, we were both confident. After five kilometres, I lost him – but I wasn't too worried. In the last two kilometres I saw him, just ahead. I was gaining on him quickly.

He looked exhausted. 'You've got only one-and-a-half to go', I shouted as I passed. He looked surprised and lengthened his stride. We came in together, ahead of our target.

'What happened?' I asked him, later in the pub.

'The start was so easy I quit pacing myself and just went for it. Good job you caught me'.

Old habits die hard. If you really want to change, sometimes it helps to have help. And food and exercise habits are tough. Once your body knows you're listening to it again, you've got a better chance of long-term changes. But you might consider doing the exercises with somebody else to begin with; to keep each other going until the new patterns get established.

Last Week's Food Diary And Challenges

Take a look at the **Food Diary** you started last week. How easy was it for you to keep a daily record of what you eat and drink? What sort of patterns, habits or trends did you notice? Any of the following list? You might like to write the answers to these questions in your diary.

- Are there particular times when you eat particular things?

- Do you eat more at certain times of the day?

- Where do you eat your meals (and snacks)?

- Do you eat when you're bored?

- Do you enjoy every bite?

- How fast or slowly do you eat? Compared to friends? Compared to family?

- Do you eat the same food as the people you share your meals with?

- Do you eat differently when you're alone? More? Less? Different kinds of food?

- What is your favourite meal? Is it good for you?

- Do you graze, or do you stick to three meals a day?

- How far ahead of time do you plan what you eat?

- Do you enjoy your food as much as you did ten years ago? More? Less?

- Do you eat as much as you did ten years ago? More? Less?

- Does your favourite food make you happy? While you're eating it? Afterwards?

- Is there something you can't resist?

- Do you have any activities that trigger you to eat?

- Can you imagine living without your favourite food for six weeks?

- Which meal have you enjoyed the most in the last seven days? What was good about it?

- How much time do you spend thinking about food?

- How much time do you spend preparing food?

- What food feels best in your stomach after you've eaten it?

- What food smells best before you eat it?

- How well can you picture in your mind your ideal self?

- Have you noticed how active you are?

- Are you honouring your decision to change?

How Are You Doing?

It is estimated that 99% of the people who buy a book don't read past the first chapter – so you are very unusual and also very likely to succeed.

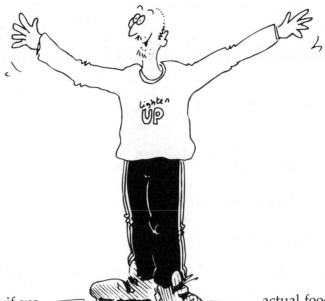

Food can be a bad habit if we use it like the other drugs we take to ease our pain. If it's another quick fix, rather than a lingering sensual pleasure. If we don't take time to really savour and enjoy it. That's why it's a good idea to get to know your own eating patterns and understand what they mean to you.

Eating tends to be an automatic process often done without much appreciation. We sometimes eat without really thinking about it. So, not only do we not know when to stop, we probably aren't getting as much enjoyment from eating as we should.

What a waste of an opportunity for pleasure!

I want you to know about every mouthful you take. I want you to enjoy every mouthful instead of ignoring it at the time and suffering a lot of grief afterwards; over something you never even tasted!

Many dieters spend hours before every meal thinking about what they are allowed (or not allowed) to eat. The actual food allowance is then eaten, almost unnoticed, in a few minutes. It's often not what they wanted to eat, or when they wanted to eat it anyway.

In the next few weeks you will be heightening your awareness because awareness is the key to unlocking change. There is no point in changing your behaviour until you know exactly what you want to change and what you want to do more often.

You will find yourself developing a big picture of your habits as you begin to become more aware of eating and of being more active every day. With the picture in front of you, it's easier to see what needs changing.

Take the time to go through the questions on the left-hand side quite slowly, and, as you write down the answers, you'll become more and more aware of your eating patterns.

Good Luck.

Common Eating Patterns

Do you recognise any of these? Tick the boxes that look familiar.

Skipping breakfast ❑

Skipping breakfast and then having a doughnut and coffee mid-morning ❑

Eating on the go ❑

Eating in the car ❑

Eating to stay awake at the computer ❑

Eating too much of one or two particular types of food ❑

Eating something sugary late afternoon ❑

Eating just to soak up the beer ❑

Ordering takeaways when you're too tired to cook ❑

Skipping meals altogether ❑

Substituting sweet or fatty snacks for meals ❑

Eating while watching TV ❑

Deciding it's easier to grab a biscuit than peel an orange ❑

Eating the biggest meal of the day late in the evening when the most strenuous activity will be picking up the remote control ❑

Eating when you're bored, angry, sad, happy or excited. ❑

Eating for any reason other than hunger. ❑

Are there any other patterns that you have?

Which one of these could you change?

Handfuls Of Pleasure

When I first met Mo, I could guarantee that if I called on her while she was watching *EastEnders* I'd find her with one of those big bags of Kettle Chips in her hand. When I teased her and tried to steal some she'd just snatch them away and say, 'Leave me alone, it's my half an hour of guaranteed pleasure at the end of a hard day'. They made her feel good. Until I messed things up by encouraging her to start tasting every mouthful.

She noticed that the first two or three handfuls were pretty good. Then there were eight or nine handfuls in between which she paid little attention to. The last few handfuls were good again because she realised her pleasure was almost finished. As she tossed the bag in the bin she often felt dissatisfied, fat or full. She asked herself why she'd eaten them in the first place.

Eventually she decided that the eight or nine handfuls in the middle of the bag were needless calories and bought some clothes pegs. If you fold over the top of the bag and clip it with a clothes peg, they still taste okay the next day.

Everybody has their patterns. Whether it's popcorn at the pictures (regardless of whether you're having a pizza afterwards) or a Crunchie bar while you're waiting for the train after work, we all have our habits. And often that's all they are, habits, not hunger.

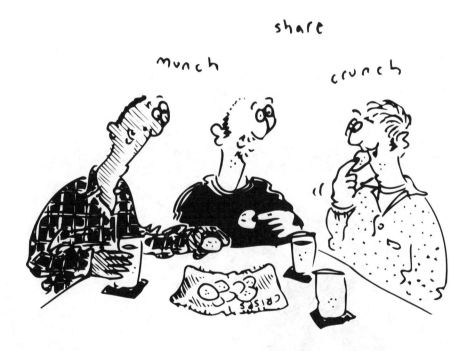

Remember, calories should be tasted, not wasted. You could always share that packet of pork scratchings.

*If you don't know what
you're doing*

today,

*how do you know
if you're going to do
something* different

tomorrow?

~ Blake Wilder, jun.

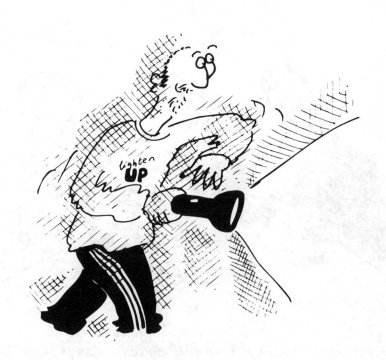

Have You Cleaned Your Teeth Today?

Many of the things we do are automatic. And that's the way they ought to be. Did you hear about the millipede that stopped to work out which leg to move next? Apparently it never did get going again. Breathing is just one of many functions that our subconscious manages very well without conscious interference, and digestion is another. But some activities we hand over to our subconscious might work better if we monitored them more closely.

An old lady once told me that she'd reached the stage where she could never remember whether she'd cleaned her teeth or not after breakfast. So, when she wasn't sure, she'd check the toothbrush. If it was wet, she knew she'd brushed them and if it was dry, she hadn't. It was usually wet.

I suppose after a lifetime of doing something it's bound to become hard-wired. And we programme in bad habits very quickly – eating patterns in particular. Like eating at lunchtime whether we're hungry or not, reaching for the biscuit tin when we get home from work, having a pudding because everybody else is.

Are you aware of any habits that might be stopping you from becoming slimmer?

Diets encourage us to take on new habits for the period of the diet itself, but most people return to familiar ways when it's finished. It's no good relying on a diet to change your life. You can only do that by changing yourself first.

One of the most common patterns is eating when we're not physically hungry. When we do this our bodies just store the food we don't need as fat. By learning how to change this you'll gain so much more control.

If you need some tools to help you with these changes, you could start with the **Hunger Scale** at the end of this chapter.

More Pink Elephants

This is part two of the **Pink Elephant** exercise from last week. It takes practice. Most people find it much easier to define what they want to avoid. Like WEIGHT. Presumably that's why they join classes to watch it. It's not surprising the weight won't go away if it's on your mind all the time.

What do you want?
Go for positive answers. Instead of writing 'I must lose weight', try something like:
            'I want to be slim/healthy/fit/beautiful.'

What will that do for you?
What benefits might you gain from whatever it is you want? For example, being fit might mean you can go swimming and feel good in a bikini, or wear short skirts again.

How will you know that you've got what you want?
What changes might happen in your life as a result of getting whatever it is that you want? Where would you be spending more time? What would you be doing that you aren't doing now?

What will you see when you get what you want?
This is the picture of you. What would you look like? Make it three-dimensional. Twirl around a little, look in the mirror. What are you wearing?

What would you feel?
Would you glow? Would you feel warm and satisfied? Cool and in control? Happy, excited, loved, interested, glamorous, confident?

What would you hear?
You might hear someone special paying you a compliment, it might just be a voice in your own head telling you how great you look. Does that ever happen? Well, it could.

See how you would look, feel how you would feel, if you were the way you want to be.
Put it all together and make a movie of the new you. Give it a soundtrack. Make yourself the star. Take some time making it really convincing. Be sure it delights you.

This, by the way, will take more practice for some people than for others.
But with plenty of practice everybody can win an Oscar.

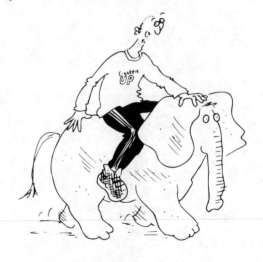

A Widescreen Technicolor Expert

Everybody daydreams. Some people are better at it than others but whether it comes naturally or not, you can become a widescreen, Technicolor expert if you concentrate. Yes, I'm actually saying you need to work harder at your daydreaming technique.

Think of an architect, or an artist. What makes the great architects and artists better than the rest? Their ability to visualise the result they want to achieve. Once they have a clear picture in front of their eyes, not too far away and very clear and bright, they are more than halfway to achieving that result.

What about some of the greatest inventors and innovators?

Take Einstein, for example. When he came up with $E = mc^2$ he wasn't poring over equations in black and white. He was imagining what it would be like to travel on a light beam. Our imaginations are grossly neglected considering how extremely useful they can be as tools for change. Most of us only use them for recreational purposes – or for upsetting ourselves if we happen to be the worrying kind.

When we were at school, looking out of the window, seeing ourselves as heroes and heroines in some wild and daring adventure, the teachers would tell us to stop it. They would tell us to look down at our books. Daydreaming was discouraged and imagination was a waste of time. Yet, if you speak to successful people (who often didn't do too well at conventional education) they will tell you how they used to dream. Steven Spielberg knew from an early age that he was going to make not just regular movies but blockbusters because he'd done it in his imagination so many times.

You get what you focus on.

Psychologists believe that, in order really to fix something in your mind, you need to repeat it twenty times. You can do the exercises on page 26 twenty times (not all at once), but there's nothing to stop you doing it thirty or forty times if you like. The more you practise, the more likely you are to get what you want.

Most people see themselves as they think they are. If you want to be successful, see yourself as you would like to be. It's the first step to getting there.

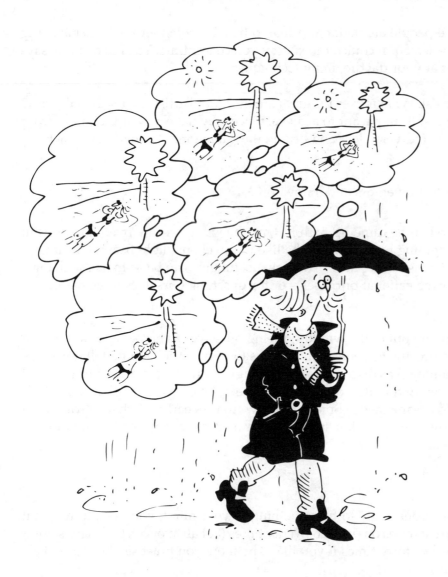

What we

VIVIDLY IMAGINE,

ARDENTLY DESIRE,

ENTHUSIASTICALLY ACT UPON,
must
INEVITABLY
come to pass.
COLIN P. SISSON

Using Your brain for a change.
– Richard Bandler

If you truly decide to, you can do almost anything. But in order to succeed, you need a strong, positive, long-term goal. Your brain will go for whatever you focus on. And, since most people focus on what they want to avoid, it's not surprising that that's exactly what they get.

Take weight for example. We spend more time thinking about the weight we want to lose than about how good we'll look when we've lost it. We spend more time worrying about things that could go wrong than anticipating good times ahead. *Looking forward* is something children do before Christmas and birthdays. *Worrying about what might happen* is something adults do all the time.

As my friend, Lisa, once said, 'There's no point in looking forward to something nice – you don't need to practise having fun, do you? It's the horrible things you keep going over in your mind because you hope by doing that, you'll be able to cope when it happens.'

I remember getting really cross with her. 'Honestly, Lisa, have you ever wondered why you don't enjoy parties and holidays as much as you used to? You're the world's expert at expecting the worst so it's hardly surprising that it's what you usually get. You wouldn't want to waste all that preparation, would you?'

It says a lot for Lisa that she's still talking to me. After all, she's not unusual.

What are the most popular TV programmes? The soaps and the disasters. The more catastrophes per hour it seems, the higher the ratings. We are all fascinated by misfortune but then we wonder why we're feeling anxious and pessimistic.

It's the same with weight. Overweight people think about their extra pounds all the time and the body generally follows what's in the mind. If you spend time trying to starve or over-exercise your body while your brain is still playing the 'fat person' video, of course, you're going to fail.

Why not start planning for success? If disasters happen, you'll cope anyway. It's the positive **Outcomes** that you need to plan for. Once you've practised some positive anticipation a few times, your brain gets a much clearer image of where you want to go.

All the greatest achievers of the twentieth century, from Edison to Branson, started being successful in their minds. Take a moment to think of something you've achieved yourself – and how you did it. And make a note of it in your diary. You might make a special section at the end, away from the **Food Diary** for this kind of information.

It's Only Words

Use three different coloured pens for this exercise:
- Underline words you associate with dieting in the first colour.
- Underline words you associate with being overweight in another colour.
- Underline words you associate with being slim and attractive in the third colour.

Achievement	Diet	Guilt	Obsession	Sweets
Anorexia	Difficult	Gymnasium	Old	Swimsuit
Anti-social	Dinner	Happy	Pain	Tablets
Anxiety	Discipline	Hard	Party	Target
Appetite	Doctors	Healthy	Pleasure	Taste
Ashamed	Drinking	Heavy	Popularity	Tea
Attraction	Drugs	Hedonism	Poverty	Temporary
Attractive	Dynamic	Hips	Pregnancy	Temptation
Beauty	Eating	Holiday	Promise	Temptress
Bed	Eating Disorder	Hollow	Psychiatry	Thin
Binge	Elegant	Home	Psychology	Tight-Assed
Bonny	Embarrassment	Hopeless	Regular Meals	Tired
Bony	Empty	Hot	Salad	Tomorrow
Boring	Endorphins	Hypnotism	Scales	Treadmill
Boy	Energy	Ill	School	Trial
Bulge	Enjoy	Image	Secret	Unfit
Bulimia	Excitement	Impossible	Security	Vegetables
Burden	Exhaustion	Insecurity	See-Saw	Vitality
Burn	Failure	Lettuce	Self-Delusion	Vitamins
Cakes	Family	Life	Self-Esteem	Waist
Calorie	Fashion	Light	Sensuality	Warm
Calorie Counter	Fast	Lonely	Sex	Wealth
Cheating	Feeling Good	Love	Sex Appeal	Weekend
Chocolate	Film Star	Lunch	Shape	Weighing
Choice	Firm	Lycra	Shopping	Weight
Christmas	Fit	Lying	Size	Winter
Clinic	Fitness	Magazines	Skin Problems	Women
Clothes	Fitting In	Martyr	Sleep	Work
Club	Flirting	Mature	Slim	Worry
Comfort	Food	Measuring	Slow	Wrinkles
Confidence	Fridge Magnets	Men	Smell	Young
Couch Potato	Friends	Milkshake	Smoking	
Counting	Fruit	Mirror	Snack	
Cottage Cheese	Fry-Up	Misery	Social	
Cuddly	Full	Model	Stable	
Dancing	Fun	Monstrous	Starving	
Date	Girl	Mother	Substitute	
Denial	Glamour	Motivation	Success	
Depression	Glow	Muscles	Suffering	
Deprivation	Grapefruit	New Year	Summer	
Deserving	Grill	Nutrition	Sweat	

Painful Experience

So words don't carry much weight?

What sort of words did you associate with dieting and being fat? Were they more, or less attractive than the words you associated with being slim and looking good?

Most people, whether naturally slim or not, associate pain and misery with dieting, and unhappiness with being overweight. So if you think you are overweight and you focus a lot on your spare tyre and the need to diet, you are going to be pretty depressed about the whole thing.

And if you are one of the many who associate exercise, love handles and diets with pain, deprivation and a downturn in your social life – don't despair. You've just been doing the wrong sort of exercise, eating the wrong food and focusing on too much pain. It's not surprising you didn't stick with it for long. You'd have to be crazy to succeed.

In fact, I'm amazed at how many people manage to hang in with complicated, anti-social, fun-free diets for as long as they do. Not only are they depriving themselves of many pleasures, but they are also often hungry which creates a painful feeling in the body. Yet, even though people have these painful perceptions, they still diet.

And you can diet forever, if you have a will of steel and low social expectations. But you can't get away from the sheer deliciousness of chocolate mousse, strawberry shortcake and sticky toffee pudding. Every now and again, or even more often than that, a treacle tart is going to creep up on you. And there's nothing wrong with treacle tart once in a while. The fat problem happens when all you can think about is treacle tart and you don't get any joy out of a banana – or a cucumber sandwich.

Your associations are related to your previous experiences, so what did you discover about your perceptions of dieting from the exercise on the previous pages?

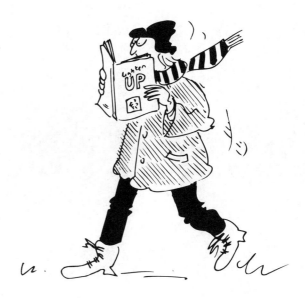

Looking For A Good Time

How do you get pleasure?

- ❤ Cooking food
- ❤ Drinking alcohol
- ❤ Eating chocolate
- ❤ Eating takeaways
- ❤ Going to parties
- ❤ Going to the cinema
- ❤ Listening to music
- ❤ Long walks
- ❤ Looking after children
- ❤ Looking good
- ❤ Playing football
- ❤ Surfing the Internet
- ❤ Reading novels
- ❤ Shopping
- ❤ Smoking
- ❤ Spending time with friends
- ❤ Taking drugs
- ❤ Watching films
- ❤ Watching football
- ❤ Watching the TV
- ❤ Exercising
- ❤ Dancing
- ❤ Cycling

What are the long-term effects of your favourite activities?

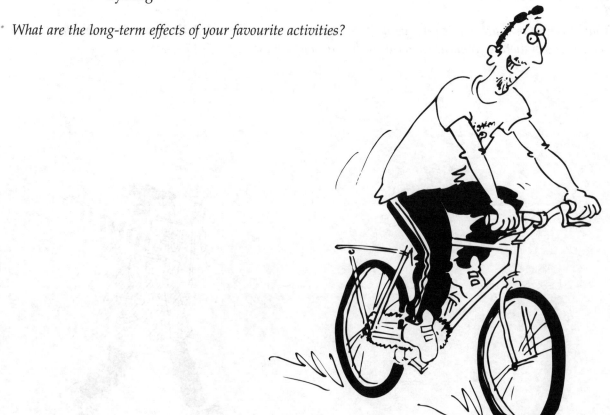

Exercising Your Right To Pleasure

Go back to the word list: take a quick look over it with the idea of exercise rather than dieting in mind. Which words jump out at you now?

There are some people who feel the adrenaline surge just by thinking about going for a swim or a run or a step class. But a lot of people don't.

I have always been amazed by how many people hate the idea of exercise. They think it's going to hurt. They know they are going to hate it so they set out to prove themselves right.

Expecting it to be hell, we often start a new slimming programme by exercising daily at way above our personal limits. The self-fulfilling prophecy strikes again. After a few weeks of painful workouts, it's no wonder we often go back to the pleasures we miss, the comfort we've denied ourselves and a happy, lardy life.

I believe that everything we do is governed by our perception of whether our actions will lead to pleasure or pain. It's as if we have a biological mechanism inside us that constantly looks to avoid pain and gain pleasure. We want pleasure in the moment and so we go for the quick fix, eating fattening foods, smoking, drinking or taking other drugs.

Quick-fix dependency is an epidemic. You can buy a fix for the way you feel. But the quicker the fix, the more likely there is to be long-term damage: heart disease, cancer. Think ahead.

Many of my clients have eaten food to change the way they feel, even though they knew they'd feel full, fat, guilty and uncomfortable when they finished eating. Yet, the pleasure of the anticipation and the moment of eating, is a stronger hit than the pain that follows. But it needn't be that way.

Do you think dieting is painful? Or being hungry? Or exercising?

I have some ideas that could change things for you. Firstly, what about learning to eat when you're hungry instead? Believe me, it's a great feeling compared to eating when you aren't really hungry. And, if you learn to finish before you're too full, you won't even get any painful feelings when you've finished your meal.

The next thing I'll be teaching you is how to change your perceptions so that you start associating pleasure with being more active and pain with being inactive. You can start the process now by thinking about all the pleasure you'll get from being slimmer, fitter and healthier.

The Exercise Wheel

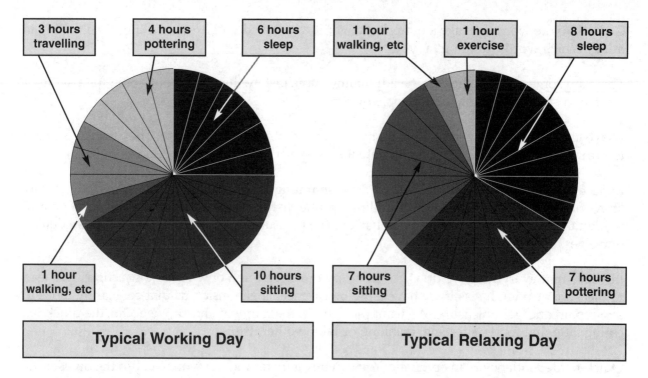

Sleeping
Sitting: working at a desk or VDU, eating, watching TV, travelling
Pottering about: light housework, office work, shopping
Walking/cycling/stairs/escalators: going somewhere fast without breaking a sweat
Travelling: driving or public transport
Exercise: sport, aerobics, circuit training, running, dancing

Each segment is an hour of the day. Colour in your typical activity pattern on a working day and a weekend/day off, using different colour or shading for each of the five categories.

See if you can change your pattern over the next couple of weeks and change the balance on your two wheels.

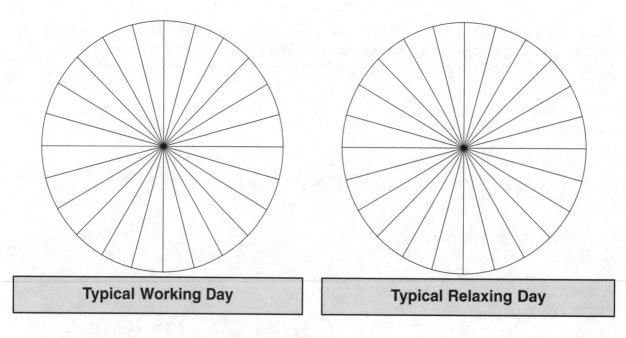

The Missing Link

A few weeks ago I volunteered to help a friend of mine organise some games for her little boy's birthday party. I hadn't been in a confined space with so many five-year-olds since I was at school myself. After an hour I was exhausted. The energy levels at that party were higher than the toughest aerobic class I've ever led. I'd forgotten how children run around all the time. They are constantly in motion. Which is why you don't see so many overweight children as over-weight adults. (Though there are more now than there used to be, because they don't seem to walk to school and play out in the street any more.)

Our bodies are designed to do one thing and one thing only. MOVE. The fuel that powers them is FAT. And, if we don't use our bodies today, the fuel gets stored for tomorrow. Which never comes.

We drive to work. We take the lift to the second floor as well as the twenty-second. We sit down in front of a screen all day; then we go home and sit down in front of a screen all evening, pausing only to order a pizza when we think we ought to be hungry. Fitting in the average twen-ty-six hours of television a week viewing doesn't leave much time for dancing, cooking or even taking the kids out to play games. No wonder so many of us complain of feeling tired all the time.

The environment we live in does nothing to encourage activity. We don't have to work the land or chase our food – we can even order groceries on the Internet and have them delivered if we really don't want to shake out too many fat cells before we stock up the larder again.

So we don't get much exercise out of necessity and most of us don't go out and exercise for fun either. PE at school cured us of that and the association with discomfort, humiliation and goosebumps lingers on. And slogans like *No Pain No Gain* and *Go For The Burn* reinforced the general aversion. So how does someone like me go about convincing people that fat-burning exercise is comfortable and fun?

The answer is *pleasure*. I believe that's what motivates us all and out there, somewhere, is a fun form of exercise for everybody. An enjoyable, comfortable activity is the best way to break up fat cells. You can be active enough without ever moving out of your comfort zone, and the great thing is that normally active people burn fat even while they watch television.

My **Outcome** for this book is to convince you that exercise and activity are the most powerful, natural and happy ways to live a healthy life.

In fact, I'd like to suggest that you put this book down now and go for a short, brisk walk. If you hear yourself saying: *'I can't, I haven't got time, I'm tired'*, just tell yourself to *'shut up'*, and think about how good you'll feel when you're actually walking and how wonderful you'll feel when you go to bed tonight with a tired body as well as an exhausted mind.

The Hunger Scale

Hunger is the only good reason for eating. Most overweight people have got into the habit of eating when they are not hungry.

Using the **Hunger Scale** is a great habit breaker because you will start to ignore your normal eating triggers and learn to recognise a new one – HUNGER. Your relationship with food will improve as you begin to notice how hungry you are.

Ask yourself before you eat, 'How hungry am I on a scale of 1 to 10?'

If you register 6, 7 or 8, you're probably quite hungry so it's time to eat.

If you score 9 or 10 this is extreme hunger. When you're eating at this level take it slowly.

If you register 5 or below, you are more than likely not hungry. And, if you're not hungry, what are you? What else would hit the spot for you right now?

Record the figure on your food sheet.

1	2	3	4	5	**6**	**7**	**8**	9	10
Not Hungry				Fairly Hungry		Where you want to be			Starving

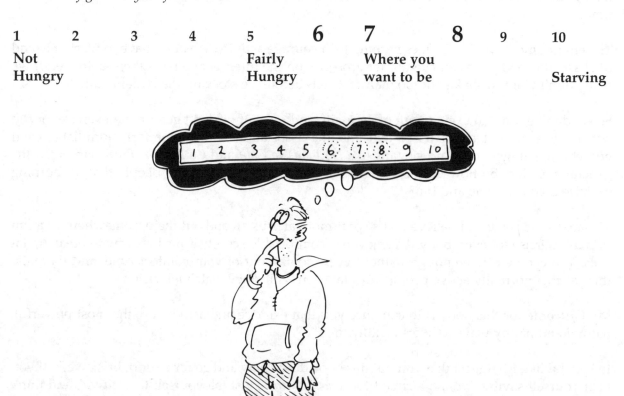

Diets imply that we are unable to manage our bodies and our eating. A lot of people go along with this because they love the security of a diet. They're afraid of eating for pleasure and they've forgotten how to eat when they're hungry. Most diets tell you to ignore pleasure and ignore hunger and they also tell you when, how much and exactly what to eat. It's like being a baby again. We have lost touch with our natural responses to physical and emotional needs. My goal is to teach you how to listen to yourself, instead of living by a set of somebody else's rules.

Planning To Eat

Many conventional diets contain a lot of common sense, although some of them are downright dangerous. The problem with most of them is that they don't teach you to be self-reliant and listen to your own body. They teach you to stick to a formula and live by the book. A lot of diets encourage dieters to be even more obsessional than they are already. Focusing on mealtimes, counting calories, weighing portions of food, weighing yourself, making a big deal out of a daily or weekly treat.

The only way you will ever lose weight is by getting back in touch with what your own body needs and learning to enjoy food and exercise all over again.

Diets overlook a crucial question. Dieters can get so caught up with following the diet that they never actually ask themselves **that** question:

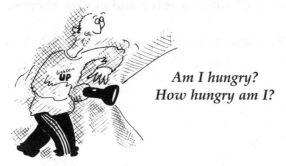

Am I hungry?
How hungry am I?

I've seen people force themselves to eat their two-hundred calorie snack on the dot of 11.30am when they weren't hungry at all. But they had to do it because the diet said so. Then, when they were starving two hours later, they were allowed only the grapefruit and spinach salad.

If you eat when you are not hungry, your body will turn *whatever you eat* into fat.

If you don't eat when you are hungry, your body thinks it's being starved and uses your muscles for fuel and energy, hanging on to the precious fat reserves for when things get really tough.

Trust me. No, trust yourself. You don't need a diet to tell you when to eat and how much.

Your body can tell you that.

Measuring Your Success

How will you know you are getting slimmer if you don't weigh yourself?

As you become more aware of your eating patterns, as you get used to using the **Hunger Scale**, as you become more active, you will *feel* slimmer.

- **Your clothes will feel looser.**

- **You will have more energy.**

- **You will be more active.**

- **You will be looking forward to the *Challenges* at the end of each chapter.**

- **You will be keeping a Food Diary and noticing patterns in your life that will give you the vital clues to change.**

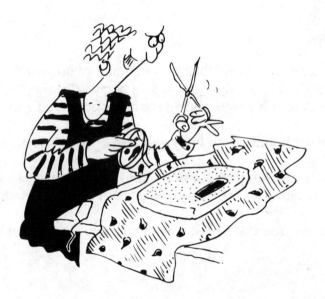

Give your scales to someone you don't like.

Off The Scales

When Lisa moved flats, she deliberately left her scales behind. A week later, the girl who moved into her old place called round to see her. She had a couple of pot plants and the scales in a carrier bag. 'You left these behind,' she said. 'Oh, and by the way, those scales are useless, I nearly threw them out – but you don't need to weigh yourself anyway, do you?'

Lisa told me the story herself, then she said, 'I feel so cross about all those bad days I had when I'd gained a couple of pounds. I remember thinking my weight was fluctuating a lot.' Then she looked at me and shook her head. 'Don't even think about saying it.'

'I told you so,' I said.

Dieters tend to rely on their oldest friend and worst enemy – the scales – to tell them how well they are doing and how much weight they've lost.

But, when you get on your scales, however accurate and high tech they are, they are not just weighing fat. They are weighing everything else as well: muscle, bone, skin and water. All of these can vary, but although most people don't mind increasing muscle and bone density they still worry about it when it shows up on the scales.

Weighing is a ritual for many people I know. They weigh themselves in the same way that they eat – automatically – without thinking about it. Lisa went through a phase of weighing herself first thing every morning, and the reading on the scales governed how she felt for the rest of the day. If there was a loss, she felt great. Half a pound too much and her day was ruined.

Your weight can change for so many biological reasons. Women retain more fluid at some times of the month than at others. Nobody can be sure about their muscle mass and tone or their exact weight distribution. I have worked with hundreds of people who have been getting gradually slimmer and who couldn't understand why their jeans were getting baggy but the scales didn't register any change for three, four, five, sometimes six weeks.

Don't trust the scales. Every time you get on them, you're focusing your mind on the very thing you want less of. If you can't bear to rid yourself of them, weigh yourself once every six weeks. Some people say it's harder to stop weighing themselves daily than to give up smoking. And I believe them. There ought to be a government health warning on bathroom scales.

There are better ways of measuring your success.

Food Diary 2

Time	Food and Drinks	Activity	Hunger Scale 1 2 3 4 5 6 7 8 9 10
7.30am	1 bowl unsweetened muesli, 1 coffee with semi-skimmed milk, orange juice	None.	3
10.30am	Doughnut and black coffee	Read paper.	6
1.45pm	Soup, wholemeal roll, apple, orange, banana, Diet Coke	Working.	7
6.30pm	Large Twix, 2 cups of tea	Doing crossword.	4
8.30pm	Chicken and chips, salad, grapes, handful of nuts and raisins, 3 glasses of wine, ½ pint of water	None.	6
Through day		1 litre mineral water	

*As well as noting when and what you eat, write down your number on the **Hunger Scale** as well.*

Try to eat more of your meals without doing anything else at the same time. But if you *are* doing something else, record that too.

munch
munch

Next Week's Diary

You should be several pages into your diary by now. You did buy yourself a notebook, didn't you?

- As you continue to write down everything you eat and drink in the **Food Diary**, you'll become increasingly aware of your eating patterns.

- Start consciously looking for patterns as you become more aware of how, when and what you eat. You might even find that you are changing some habits you never even knew you had.

- As you copy a set of **Exercise Wheel**s for the week and fill them in every day, you'll be able to see your activity levels increasing. Nothing spectacular, just walking up stairs and to the shops more often perhaps?

- Remember, calories should be tasted, not wasted. Make a note of what tastes best.

- By using the **Hunger Scale** throughout the week you will gradually notice that you are starting to eat when you're hungry and finish when you're full.

- Write down the size of portion – large or small.

- How was the food prepared? Grilled? Raw? Sauces or dressings?

- Continue to write down what you're doing when you're eating.

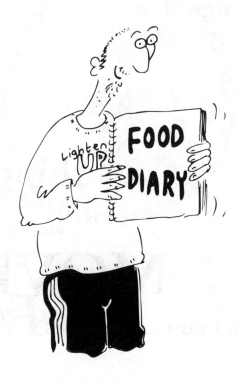

Move It And Lose It

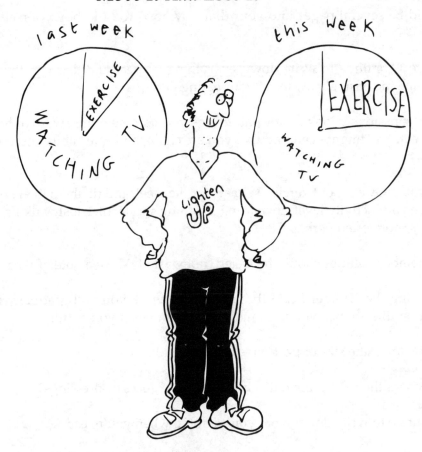

Our bodies are designed to do

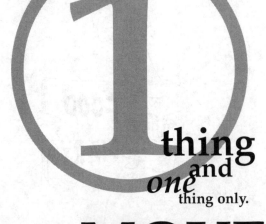

1 thing and one thing only.

MOVE.
FAT.

The fuel that powers them is *FAT.*

➡ Continue to honour your decision to change.

➡ Do all the exercises on the left-hand pages this week.

➡ Throw the scales away or donate them to a jumble sale. You could even give them to someone you don't like – making a present of bathroom scales is an excellent way of causing offence and can end a negative relationship quickly and painlessly (for you).

➡ Change at least one of your eating patterns.

➡ Think about what you want to see, hear and feel when you reach your ideal weight. Believe it and you'll achieve it.

➡ Use the **Hunger Scale**.

➡ Add more activity to your **Exercise Wheel** and make a note of it.

➡ Take the time to enjoy every mouthful of food.

➡ Look at the food section at the back of this book and have a go at one of the recipes or some of the other ideas.

➡ Look at what gives you pleasure in life and what makes you feel good.

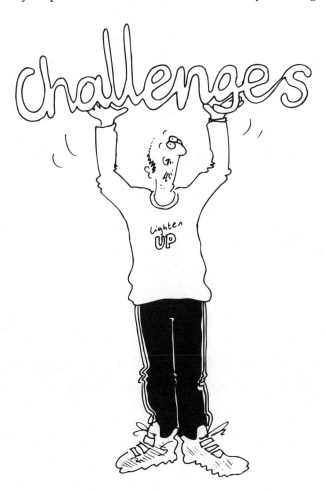

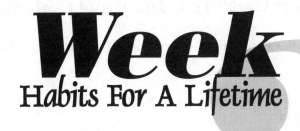

Week
Habits For A Lifetime

3

My first Lighten Up group gave me a pretty hard time. They were learning how to be slim and I was learning how they managed not to be. It was very confusing.

In the end, we all discovered the same thing. Everybody knows how to be the right size, but some of us have buried our instinctive knowledge under layers and layers of habits. And some of the habits don't even have anything to do with food.

'What are you eating that for?' I asked Lisa when she ordered black coffee and grapefruit for breakfast after an early workout. I knew she hated black coffee and grapefruit and I also knew that what she really wanted was a cappuccino and an almond croissant.

'Silly question,' she said, screwing up her face at the sharpness of the grapefruit.

'Alright then, let's re-phrase it, what did you eat last night?'

'I went to Pulchinella. You know, garlic bread, carbonara, tiramisu, coffee, those chewy almond biscuits. Plus loads of wine. Then I had a snack when I got in.'

'What was the snack for after a meal like that?' I was puzzled.

'My brother was home.'

'So?'

'Well, when we were at school he always got in before me and he always got tea ready. It's like, when we have a heart-to-heart, we always do it over a bacon sandwich at the kitchen table. He's hardly ever home now since he got posted abroad and it's kind of like nothing's changed. He sees me walk in the door and he opens the fridge.'

'I see, so it's no calories for breakfast then.'

'Are you kidding? It's no calories for the rest of the day if I want to retain any self-respect', said Lisa, bitterly.

Next time you want to tell someone you love them, DO IT.
Don't eat bacon sandwiches with them instead.

Last Week's Food Diary And Challenges

❖ Did you write up the **Food Diary** every day? It's fine if you didn't, just start again this week.

❖ As you write down how much you were eating at each meal, are you remembering to note down how it was cooked?

❖ Which good cause did you donate your scales to? I should say *'if you had any'* but I've never met a dieter who didn't. By the way, we are offering a free T-shirt to the reader with the best story about what they did with their scales – write or e-mail us, our contact details are at the end of the book.

❖ Are you still thinking about what you really want to achieve, what you'd look like and what you'd hear and feel?

❖ One thing that turns around quite quickly is the **Exercise Wheel**. Is yours looking any different to the way it was when you started? Have you increased your activity level?

❖ I expect there was at least one pattern you had a go at changing – when you changed the pattern, did it affect anything else in your life? Was it something to do with time, or a particular activity, like watching television or getting in from work?

❖ Now that you're becoming more aware of the situations or events that trigger you to eat when you aren't hungry, is this opening up new possibilities for action?

❖ Most people are surprised that the **Hunger Scale** is so easy. They always protest that it's going to be impossible, then, in their own time, they end up taking it for granted.

❖ Are you discovering new ways of getting pleasure that don't make you fat and unhealthy?

❖ Have you tried any of the recipes at the back of the book yet?

How Are You Doing?

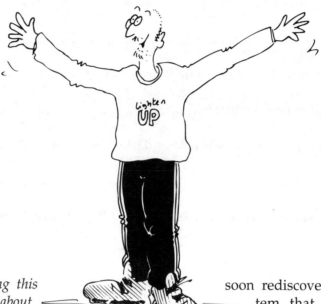

Congratulations. By reading this far, you already know a lot about what you need to do to become slimmer. The rest of the book is designed to help you practise what you've already learned at the same time as you take on the new ideas and techniques.

One of the most important ideas I introduced last week was the **Hunger Scale**. Some people look at the **Hunger Scale** and immediately know what they always knew. Others say to me, *'Well, I'm hungry all the time'*. To which I say, *'Are you really? Are you sure it isn't something else you're wanting? Company? Exercise? Distraction from a boring task? Cheering up? Waking up? A cuddle?'*

When I first introduce it, everyone always says *'How am I going to tell the difference between five and six, or seven and eight, or whatever?'* Then a couple of weeks later, they're taking it for granted. You *do* know exactly how hungry you are; you just haven't been paying attention.

I promise you, with a little practice and a lot of faith in your own intuition, you will soon rediscover the in-built system that tells you exactly what you need to keep you fit and healthy.

And, by the way, need and pleasure aren't mutually exclusive. In fact they should both be a part of your eating schedule. Eat when you need to and enjoy every mouthful.

Were you surprised by how much you ate in a day? Or how little? Most people would say they know what they eat, but it's easy to forget the odd biscuit in the afternoon or the exact number of crisps if you're sharing a bag. If it goes in your mouth it goes in the diary. There's no point in cheating on yourself, is there? Once you know what you are doing, the power to change is already in your hands.

Take the time to go slowly through the review of the **Food Diary** and the **Challenges**. It's about getting to know yourself better, and how important is that? It's about relying on yourself, rather than on someone else, to tell you how you feel and what you want.

Expecting Success

What's the difference between hoping you will be slimmer and actually expecting it to happen?

Part One

Think about what you want to achieve, whether it's wanting to be slimmer, fitter, healthier or more confident.

Write down what it is...

Close your eyes and say: *'I hope I become (whatever it is)'*

What do you see when you say that?...

What does the image look like? Is it bright or dark? How close is it?...

....

How do you *feel* when you say to yourself, *'I hope I become (whatever)'* ?.................................

....

Part Two

Now, think about what you want, but, this time, imagine that you *really expect* to become whatever it is that you want to be.

Close your eyes and say to yourself in a convincing, determined, fashion: *'I will achieve my goal. I will become ...., I expect...............'*

Repeat this a few times and notice what you see. Take the image you have and make it brighter, bolder, clearer and more real as you bring it closer towards you.

What is the difference in how you feel when you expect rather than just hope? Compare the two feelings.

Hoping is never good enough. *Expecting* gets results. Don't leave the things you really want to chance: 'It might happen, it could happen ...' Those statements have doubt built into them.

You can if you think you can.

The Successful Slimming Formula

There is a formula for becoming slimmer, fitter and healthier, just as there is a formula for the way most things operate and work in life. Sod's Law is a good example – if you drop a slice of bread it's bound to fall butter side down.

Most people want to succeed, whether in business, in life, in love or in losing weight. So why do only a few people actually manage it?

The answer is simple: they are using the wrong formula and working against nature, rather than with it.

When I first got involved with people who wanted to be slimmer, it became part of my mission to talk to as many successful slimmers as I could find. I wanted to know how they had reached the goal that seemed impossible to so many.

I believed that if I could find out what these slim people had done, what they'd eaten, what they thought about and how much exercise they had taken, I could teach their strategies to the 95% of dieters who always relapsed.

It took a while but eventually I found a totally consistent pattern which fitted all the successful slimmers. They had some specific attitudes in common, they used similar techniques and made consistent lifestyle changes. Their ability to lose weight had nothing to do with luck, dieting or having a high metabolic rate.

These people had become totally fed up with feeling fat and guilty all the time. They had started thinking specifically about what it would be like to be slim and they had increased their daily activity rate. They had also learned to associate their discomfort to over-eating in general and to large amounts of fattening and sugary foods in particular.

They learned how to enjoy the food that made them feel good and they ate only when they were physically hungry. They used their personal power to take positive action and move towards their goal.

They were passionate about changing and becoming slimmer. They had all made a committed decision to look better and be fitter and healthier and they were prepared to do whatever it took to achieve their goals. They cut themselves off from any other possibility – they *expected* to be successful. They did not hope or dream about things working out. They knew they would achieve their desired state (although some of them had *never* been slim before) and they could clearly see what it would be like.

Can you image Michael Jordan, Sally Gunnell, Madonna, Muhammad Ali, Alan Shearer or Margaret Thatcher simply hoping for success? No. They expect it, so they have no other option.

Opening Doors

Find a quiet place where you can do this exercise without being disturbed for about five minutes. You need to feel comfortable and relaxed and free from distractions. You might find the exercise easier with a friend who can talk you through these instructions so that you can disengage your conscious mind.

1. Stand up with a couple of feet of space in front of you.

2. Close your eyes and see your front door in your mind. Make it a life-size image. Imagine you are standing outside and watch your door opening.

3. Imagine now as your door opens in front of you, that you can see yourself through that door at some time in the future. You are slimmer, fitter and healthier. See yourself exactly as you want to be. You are at your ideal weight, glowing with health and feeling confident and happy.

4. Make the picture life-size and notice the firmness and clarity of your skin, the muscle and tone of your body. Make the picture so clear and bright that you could reach out and touch it. Make it vivid, colourful, and brilliant. It doesn't matter if it's not as sharp as you want it at first, because, with daily practice, your image becomes more real.

5. Now imagine the Future You, turning round right in front of you. Take a step forward into the Future You. Literally walk into your new, slim, fit and healthy body, like putting on a new skin.

6. As you do this, notice how it feels, notice how light and elegant you've become. Feel the comfort and grace of your movements as you now begin to open your eyes in the new you.

7. Pause for a moment and recognise how this changes the way you feel.

8. Take that feeling and run through the exercise again. This time double the power, make it crystal clear and see how attractive you look and feel as your confidence increases. You are the director, producer and star of your own movie so make your performance an Oscar winner.

9. Repeat this exercise every day as you come closer and closer to the Future You now.

Paul McKenna, *Slim Now*

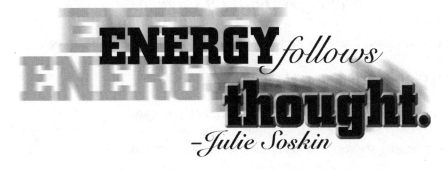

ENERGY *follows* **thought.**
–Julie Soskin

When I ask you now what you want, you are able to tell me in some detail. Your image is clear in your mind. When you see yourself in the light of how you want to be, you have all the willpower you need. You won't have to struggle with sensible eating or force yourself to be more active. The positive actions you take are moving you closer to the compelling, future, slimmer You.

You've heard the saying:

You are what you eat

... well, there's a better one:

You are what you think

Our lives are governed by our thoughts and if you think you are fat and overweight, you'll have pictures in your mind to support this. You will be building your daily life on this image – reinforcing the belief that you are fat every time you think about it. Conventional diets don't deal with people's thoughts. Maybe that's another reason why so many people regain all their weight again so soon after a diet. They still *think* they're fat. They don't know how to live thin. And slowly, the weight creeps back on to wherever they've convinced themselves it belongs.

To avoid that happening to you, use the exercise on the left. It will help you develop an even clearer positive image of yourself. Each and every time you practise that exercise, you send a message to your unconscious mind which reminds you, right now, that you are losing weight.

The Opening Doors exercise focuses your mind on your target making it more powerful and real. Every time you say 'No' to food when you're not hungry, you're saying 'Yes' to being slimmer, as you now move closer and closer to your future self. The more real the image, the less negative and judgmental you will be. You'll be turning automatically towards a stronger sense of your mission and purpose.

Thinking slim is the most important factor in achieving permanent slimness. Change your mind and you change your body as well.

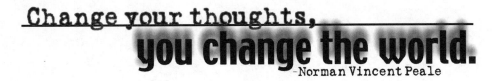

Change your thoughts, you change the world.
-Norman Vincent Peale

Making A Habit Of Change

- Always have some food available so that when you *are* hungry you can eat.

- Use the **Hunger Scale** before you eat.

- Separate eating from your other activities whenever you can.

- Replace fattening, sugary foods with fruit or other healthy snacks.

- Slow down your eating and finish when you know you've had enough. Be prepared to wait for the signal!

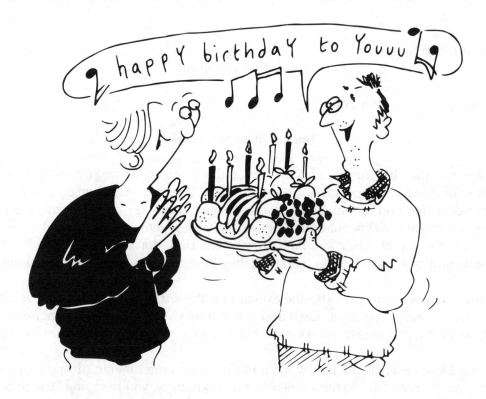

- Be open to different angles on familiar subjects. What does a fruit cake mean to you, for example?

- Include as much physical activity in your daily life as possible.

Challenging Changes

Change is definitely *possible* with determination and the right help (that's what this book is for).

Attempts to change sometimes meet the strongest resistance at the beginning. Your own body protests when you first drink tea without sugar. Then, after a while, the tea doesn't taste right with sugar in it. Other people don't like you changing either. If you don't have a Hobnob, they might feel guilty about eating one themselves. If you can get over the first hurdle, you will likely succeed.

Many of our eating patterns have been with us for years. We've been comforted and placated with food since we were too small to argue. What do you always get on your birthday? A cake, of course.

So we may have been taught to associate food with particular emotions from our earliest days. But the good news is that we can change anything we weren't born with – no matter how long we've been doing it. We don't have to be stuck with any of those learned behaviours and, with strength and determination, we can unlearn them by taking on new, empowering patterns.

Most of us like an easy, predictable life. When change seems hard, it's not so much fear of the unknown as our desire to stay inside our comfort zones that stops us. Break through and take action to change your habits. People who've succeeded in becoming slimmer usually link massive amounts of pain to slobbing out or eating lard and loads of pleasure to being active, fit and slender.

Can you control pain and pleasure? Of course you can. But you can only start the process by taking decisive action, which may be uncomfortable at the beginning. The challenge is to use pain and pleasure instead of pain and pleasure using you. That's the secret of success. If you do this you will be in control of your life. If you don't, then life controls you.

Use your power to follow through. Every time you take appropriate action, like walking to the shops or eating when you're hungry, you are becoming more and more powerful.

Change is happening in and around us all the time. We grow new cells, we learn new ideas, the seasons turn and the weather is never what you expect. So open up to change and changes will happen.

Challenge Yourself

Some of these questions may get familiar answers, but there will be some surprises too.

Give all the questions your equal attention and write down the answers. It will be like a roller coaster because we are switching between pain and pleasure.

- What pain and discomfort do you associate with changing your diet and increasing your exercise level?

- What pleasure have you got from eating what you want and being inactive?

- What will it cost you if you don't become more active and eat a better, healthier diet?

- What would you like to be like in the future? Would you be slimmer? How would you look? What sort of clothes would you be wearing? The **Open Door** exercise you've just done is great for strengthening this image.

- How would you feel about yourself if you were slimmer, fitter and healthier?

- List all the pleasure you'll get from being slimmer, fitter and healthier.

- What will you gain?

- How will you look and feel?

- How will your life be different?

The Secret

THE SECRET OF SUCCESS
is learning how to use pain and pleasure instead of pain and pleasure using you. If you do that, you're in control of your life. If you don't, life controls you. *— Anthony Robbins*

It's hard for many of us because, intellectually, we know that eating fattening foods and leading a sedentary life is bad for us. We often try to change, but all those years of fast food and slow moves weigh us down. We instinctively flinch from the prospect of long-term change.

And, of course, we often share our lives with people who have a similar lifestyle to our own and who may be in similar shape. If we change, they may feel worse about themselves – so we aren't likely to get much support from them. Or perhaps we're surrounded by slim, fit and beautiful people. It doesn't matter. They are used to us being the way we are. When we change, *they* find it more threatening than we do. Because we already made the effort and the decision whereas they are probably taken by surprise. We said so many times before that we were going to do things differently. But we never did – until now.

If you speak to the people who have lost weight and kept if off, they will often tell you that the thought of exercising and eating well used to be painful to them – until, one day they turned that perception on its head. *Now* they find the thought of endless chips and chocolate quite painful because they know how fat and full they are going to feel afterwards. They've also learned to enjoy being active and they hate the thought of missing out on the exercise they have made a part of their daily routine.

You have already started this process. Now is the time to associate more pleasure with that image of yourself you will be building for the future.

As you answer the questions on the left-hand side, you can start to understand some of the reasons why you are not as slim and active as you would like to be. And at the same time you can allow yourself to start feeling the pleasure of the changes you are beginning to make.

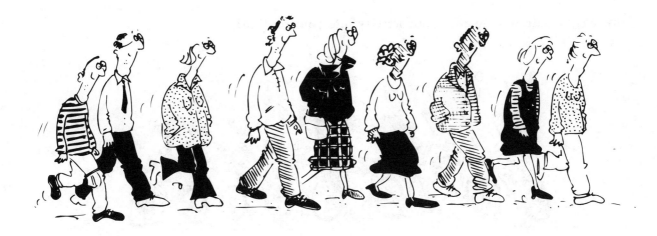

The 5% Solution

THESE FOLKS HAVE FOUND THE SECRET OF BEING ABLE TO INCORPORATE *EXERCISE* INTO THEIR LIVES. DR JIM HILL, CO-DIRECTOR OF THE NATIONAL WEIGHT LOSS REGISTRY, DESCRIBING A STUDY OF THE 5% OF PEOPLE WHO MAINTAINED A THIRTY POUNDS WEIGHT LOSS FOR MORE THAN A YEAR.

When you start filling in your **Exercise Wheel** regularly, you can get a better impression of whether you are getting enough exercise. Human beings weren't designed to spend most of their lives sitting down.

Lots of things we take for granted count as good exercise. And you can add in activities which are extremely good in terms of turning up your metabolic thermostat, but which needn't involve complicated arrangements at the gym or the squash court – unless you want them to.

How many of the following activities do you already do and how many could you add?

Activity

	Already do it?	Times per week?	Add it?
Walking to work	❑	❑	❑
Walking part of the way to work	❑	❑	❑
Walking to the shops/school	❑	❑	❑
Recreation involving exercise	❑	❑	❑
Cycling instead of other transport	❑	❑	❑
Walking up stairs and escalators	❑	❑	❑
Running up stairs	❑	❑	❑
Getting up hourly at work and stretching	❑	❑	❑
Mini-stretch programme while watching TV	❑	❑	❑
Housework	❑	❑	❑
Gardening	❑	❑	❑
Outdoor games with children	❑	❑	❑
Walking a dog	❑	❑	❑
What else?	❑	❑	❑

How easy would it be to add more activity into your routine?

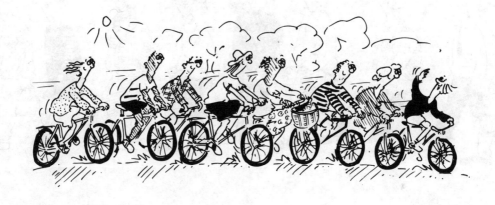

Take It Easy

As you now know, bodies were just designed to move. And if you move it you'll lose it – fat that is.

The main criterion for weight loss is that it should be continuous and steady. Aerobic exercise should always be comfortable regardless of your level of fitness. If you can't talk or whistle at the same time, you are overdoing it. If you're hating every second and feeling totally out of breath, it's because your body is failing to get oxygen to your muscles. When that happens you are working without oxygen, anaerobically. This isn't useful exercise.

Fat people get exhausted and breathless when they exercise too hard because their bodies are trying to maintain the status quo by saving fat and burning sugar (glucose). The result is painful, disheartening and doesn't result in fat reduction.

Muscles need oxygen to function and the harder they are worked the more oxygen they need. But hard doesn't mean painful. Aerobic exercise simply means exercise that uses oxygen. Any vigorous activity like cleaning or gardening is aerobic so you don't *need* to go to special exercise classes. Aerobic exercise that uses the big muscles of the lower body, like cycling, walking, dancing, rowing, jogging and swimming should be kept up at a comfortable pace for a minimum of 15 minutes. The more muscles incorporated into an exercise, the better.

As you get into the habit of becoming more active, your shape will start to change, you'll feel healthier – and you might wonder how you managed without those good feelings you get from steady, regular exercise.

The best way to get back to your natural blueprint is to use your body for what it was made to do.

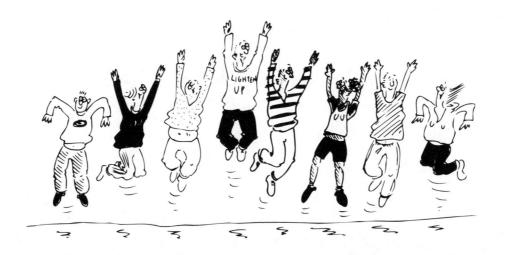

Move It And Lose It

The Fat Jar

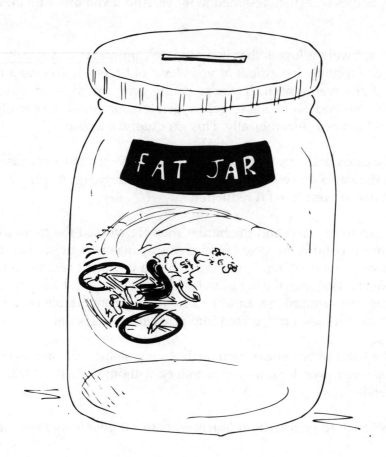

Be A Fat-burning Machine, Not A Fat-storing Machine

Fifteen minutes of continuous activity seems to be the time trigger necessary to stimulate production of fat-burning enzymes. The more of these you have, the more fat you can burn. But although it takes fifteen minutes to start the enzymes increasing, the ones you already have will be burning fat for you from the very first step you take.

Get yourself a jar. Every time you walk briskly for fifteen minutes, put a five pence piece in it. That way you can *see* how active you are and how much more active you are becoming. You might want actually to imagine the fat from your body going into the jar. On the other hand, that is pretty gross, so feel free not to imagine it.

What's the difference between just burning fat and growing more fat-burning enzymes? It's like the difference between burning logs in the fireplace you already have and enlarging that fireplace so that you can burn more at a time. If your fireplace is already big enough, that's fine. But fat people have smaller fireplaces and only burn small logs. The more exercise you do over the next weeks and months, the bigger your fireplace becomes and the more fat logs you can burn.

It's not about counting calories. That's as depressing and obsessional as counting the calories you eat. Forget about it. Calorie-burning is the least important part of exercise. The main purpose of becoming more active is to become efficient at using fat for your major energy source instead of storing it.

The main criterion for exercise is that it should be comfortable and continuous.

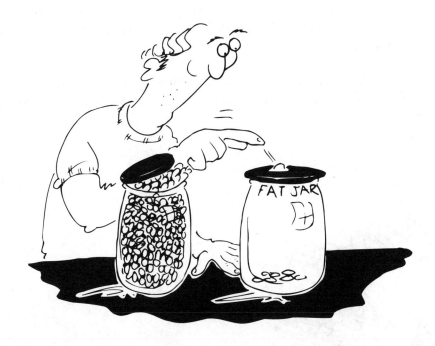

Think Before You Eat

Something makes you think of food. You might look at your watch and notice that it's lunchtime, hear the word *'chocolate'*, or see food. You might even feel hungry.

Whatever does it for you.

Find a quiet place where you can relax. Ask someone to read this exercise out to you (or record it yourself onto a tape). Close your eyes.

1. Now that the idea of eating has come into your mind, check whether you're getting any physical sensations or if you could be just lonely or bored.
2. If you've got some feelings that would make you think you are over 5 on the **Hunger Scale**, ask yourself what might satisfy that hunger.
3. What comes to mind? A Spam sandwich in batter with curry sauce? A banana? A slice of Battenburg?
4. Now run through the process of eating it, in your mind. Taste it, smell it, feel it in your mouth and swallow it. Imagine how you'll be feeling half an hour or so afterwards.
5. If you think you'll feel better than you do now before you've eaten, put the banana, or whatever it was, on a mental list. If you don't think a banana will see you happily through the afternoon, don't bother making a note of it.
6. Keep doing this until you've got a few choices in mind.
7. Check out your choices, one at a time, for their long-term effect on your happiness and wellbeing.
8. If you find it difficult to distinguish between *'good and satisfying'* and *'naughty but nice'* try a few deliberately wacky opposites. Like toffee crunch ice cream with treacle tart compared with a tuna salad sandwich on granary bread.

When you get fed up with doing this, or your lunchtime is running out, make a choice. Most people find, over time, that this process leads them to make more and more healthy eating decisions.

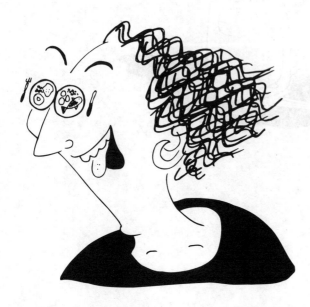

Think Before You Eat

Our stomachs contain sensory nerves that tell us when to eat and when to stop. So listen.

Relationships with food can be complex. That's why it helps to keep a diary. It's the diary of a relationship that you aren't happy with and want to change. But you need to understand it first.

There may be some benefits you get from eating that you could get, calorie-free, somewhere else. Food for comfort, food to celebrate, food to console and food for food's sake. Different events, feelings, times and trigger situations can make you feel like eating, regardless of whether you are hungry. Seeing food, or even pictures of food (which are everywhere), smelling food, seeing somebody walk past you with a hamburger. Even looking at the clock. There's no escape from the suggestion that it might be time for something to eat.

Many of the foods you eat in these situations are fattening ones that leave you feeling tired, bloated and guilty. When you ask yourself, afterwards, 'Why did I eat that?' it's too late.

The *Think Before You Eat* strategy takes a bit of practice. Like the other techniques in this book you can practise it alone or with a friend, whichever suits you. It takes a few minutes when you first start doing it, but soon, you'll zoom through it in seconds. Almost subliminally. But take it seriously, it's a powerful piece of software for re-programming your mind and body.

Remember, once you've changed your attitude you are no longer battling with yourself. Your thoughts and energy can be directed into things that make you feel happy and totally in control instead of feeling miserable and out of control.

Since working on this programme, I have talked to many slim and not-so-slim people and the thin ones almost always had their own version of **Think Before You Eat** hard-wired into their brains. In contrast, people with weight problems usually have much simpler eating strategies. They can be triggered to eat by a time of day, an activity, a feeling, an event, a person, a place – anything in fact other than hunger.

*Connirae Andreas also describes a similar technique in her book, **Heart of the Mind.** She explains that, as a naturally slim person, she based the method on her own approach to eating and has used it to help many people to lose weight easily and without stress.*

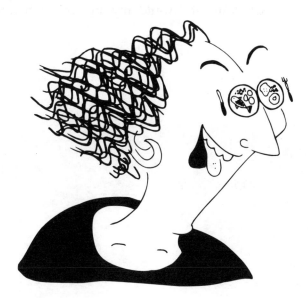

Are You Hungry?

How easily can you tell the difference between hunger and tension, or hunger and boredom?

Some Signs of Hunger

- Smelling or tasting a food you want when it's not there.

- Knowing exactly what you want to eat.

- Empty feelings in the stomach.

- Sharp, but not unpleasant sensations in the stomach, accompanied by rumbling.

- Loss of energy.

- Irritability.

- Light-headedness.

- Slightly nauseous headache accompanied by desire to eat.

- Sudden fall in motivation for the task in hand.

- Inability to think about anything but food.

- Stomach rumbling when you're not being interviewed.

*How do you know just where you are on the **Hunger Scale**? And how do you know if you're feeling hungry? Well, if you're not sure, you're probably not. Run these checks before you grab a sandwich.*

- **Think Before You Eat.**

- If you have food in front of you, smell it before tasting it.

- Ask yourself, 'Would anything other than food satisfy me at this point?'

If I'm Not Hungry, What Am I?

Everybody's different, and it's all about getting to know yourself. Before you assume that your rumbling stomach or nauseous headache means hunger, run a few double checks to help you get to know what hungry means for you:

- Bored with what you're doing and looking for something to distract you.

- Tired (eating can wake you up and give you an energy boost, but it might be better to just take a nap – or go for a walk).

- Tense or anxious – have you noticed your stomach tends to rumble or contract in interviews?

- Thirsty (may be confused with hunger, especially if the craving's for something juicy).

- Clock watching. So what if it's tea time?

- Angry – a cup of tea and a chocolate digestive are reliable sources of comfort.

- Lonely – eating's the next best thing to having company.

- Depressed – there's nothing like a piece of fudge cake to cheer you up.

- In need of comfort. Some days – and some parts of the day – can seem pretty bleak.

- Needing to chew or suck something – this is a fairly primitive one.

- Remembering good times past – this happens sometimes when you see appetising food unexpectedly.

- Suffering from indigestion (often confused with hunger pangs).

- People (usually in books) say they are *'hungry for love'*. That need really is a kind of hunger, so no wonder we try to satisfy it with food. It's a lot easier to order a takeaway than find the love of your life.

You Are What You Eat

- What does the food you eat say about you?

- Do you think you have a balanced diet?

- Does it include plenty of fresh fruit and vegetables?

- How, specifically, do the foods you eat make you feel?

- How do you prepare your food?

- What foods are you drawn towards and feel compelled to eat? Are they good for you?

- Do you know why you like some things and not others? Un-mashed tinned tomatoes in school dinners or eating a dodgy prawn can put you off some perfectly nutritious foods for life.

- Are there any foods you like the look of but have never tasted?

- Are there some foods you've never eaten but *know* you wouldn't like?

- Do you eat certain types of food at certain times of day?

- Can you smell some foods when they aren't around? Cucumber? Garlic? Melted cheese? Chips with vinegar? Chocolate? Bread? If you divided the foods you can smell without seeing into separate lists, which would be the longest? Would it be fruit and vegetables? Sweet things? Salty, savoury food?

- Look at the recipe section at the end of the book to give you ideas for a healthier diet. There are suggestions for:

  - All-day breakfasts
  - Jacket potatoes
  - Five-minute recipes
  - Sensational snacks
  - Sandwiches
  - Real food recipes
  - Fruit drinks

Over the next few weeks you'll become more aware of your patterns and associations with food and you'll start changing some of them for ever.

Healthy Diets

What do you think constitutes a healthy diet?

Your answer to this question will probably tell you that you know quite a bit about healthy diets.

Foods we eat are made up of :

- carbohydrates,
- fats,
- proteins,
- vitamins and minerals,
- water.

Our diet needs to include all of these in some form. Our bodies need them all to be able to function properly.

Dietary advice has changed many times over the past thirty years and some of the information appears to conflict. Don't give up. The key is to eat a wide variety of fresh foods from all the groups rather than cutting out one or more of them completely as so many diets seem to do.

There is no magic diet that guarantees weight loss.
Go for balance rather than perfection and eat what you enjoy. Cream slices three times a day wouldn't do, but one cream slice once in a while wouldn't be so terrible.

There is no perfect diet either.
Go for variety and balance and make sure you eat things you can enjoy – even if they aren't always chocolate-flavoured or deep-fried. Natural, fresh products are best because the human body has had years of practice at digesting them and can convert them easily into energy.

Foods that are pre-prepared and packaged are more likely to be chemically enhanced or preserved and our gut has only had a few years to get used to these new substances.

Over the next couple of weeks, I am going to suggest some simple diet strategies, which should be highly effective. You'll notice that we're nearly half-way through the book before we really start to talk about *what* you eat.

That's because I know that using the *Hunger Scale* and *Think Before You Eat*, will lead you naturally into making good food choices.

Stop, Look And Listen

Active eating means giving yourself up fully to the enjoyment of your meal. It doesn't mean being active while you're eating. The activity comes afterwards.

If you eat

- When you're watching TV

- Working

- Driving

- Speaking to someone on the phone

you're not giving food the attention it deserves.

> * Separate eating from other activities by doing nothing while you eat.

> * Remember, calories should be tasted not wasted.

If eating is a focused, orgasmic experience you will get so much more pleasure from it as you re-sensitise yourself to the signals your body naturally gives out. Signals that you might have been ignoring for some time.

You will begin to know when you've had enough and you'll have a better understanding of how food is making you feel.

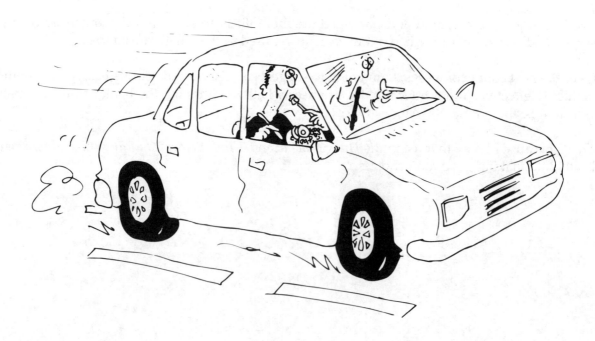

Enjoy More

Enjoy More Food or Enjoy Food More?

We often associate eating with other activities and combine it with something else. This is a shame because then we don't concentrate on eating and we often miss out on some of the pleasure we could get from it.

Since I started work on Lighten Up, I've spent a lot of time watching other people eating. Family, friends, clients, strangers in restaurants. In fact there was a time in my life when I must have been North London's least popular dinner companion. What did I notice – apart from the fact that nobody likes to be watched while they're eating? I noticed that the people who ate the most enjoyed it the least. Big eaters are often fast eaters. I'd make a comment like, 'The salsa on these nachos is a bit hot, isn't it?' and I'd look at Lewis and I'd know by the expression on his face that he hadn't even spotted there were three different kinds of sauce on his corn chips. He'd been talking about the football or looking at the woman at the next table – or whatever. But he'd been wasting his time on the nachos, he might as well have been on a drip feed.

Eating's important enough for you to give it your full attention. It's one of the great sensual pleasures of life, why rush it?

Concentrate on the taste and texture of what you're eating. Smell it first and see how appetising it is before you even put it in your mouth. If you're at a buffet or in a canteen, take time to sniff and separate out the smells before you make your choice. Don't ever decide what to eat by appearance alone.

Find out just how much pleasure you can get from your food. Set aside time to eat when your mind isn't somewhere else and your body isn't doing something else – and enjoy. Over the next few weeks, give yourself as many opportunities as possible to concentrate on eating, separating it from other activities.

If this bothers you, it's probably a sign that you are hooked on the association of eating with other activities. I know it's a cliché, but the harder it is to do this, the more you need to learn to do it.

I remember visiting Mo one night after she started becoming slimmer and the pounds started dropping off. She was watching TV, but to my amazement, she was eating an apple instead of crisps. 'Well done!' I said (patronisingly), 'Now that's what I call willpower.'

'Not really,' said Mo. 'Since I started thinking about how I feel when I'm eating, I've noticed that those Kettle Chips made me feel really thirsty and fat and depressed. They put me off my dinner and I ended up drinking beer instead. And I don't need you to tell me about the nutritional defects of lager.'

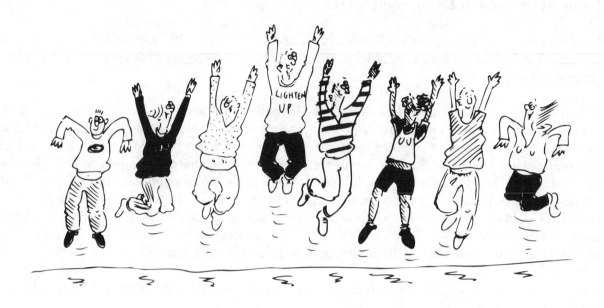

It is not because things are difficult that we do not dare;
it is because we do not dare that they are difficult.

Seneca.

Pleasures Of The Table

You might worry about your weight for lots of reasons. Maybe as you grew up you learned to use food for comfort or as an emotional crutch to change the way you felt. Maybe your family gave you food to show their love. Maybe you were always told to eat what was in front of you, never to leave food on your plate because of the starving millions or that you couldn't have any pudding if you didn't eat your meat.

Whatever the reasons for your concerns about eating, they don't matter now because you can do something about them.

If you eat when you're not hungry, your body won't respond positively by producing extra energy and making you feel good. Instead it will convert the food straight into fat for storage. Have you ever said *'I feel fat,'* when you've overeaten? That's because you're absolutely right.

Food should give us pleasure, not just from its taste and appearance but also from that injection of energy we get when we eat at more than five on the **Hunger Scale**. Concentrate on the taste and texture of what you're eating. Smell it first and see how appetising it is before you even put it in your mouth. See just how much pleasure you can get from your food. Set aside time to eat when your mind isn't somewhere else and enjoy. You can share this meal with someone else provided you agree to focus on the sensual pleasure of eating. Remember the meal in *Tom Jones*? If not, get it out on video and you'll see what I mean.

If you eat the right amount of food for you, it will not only taste a lot better than eating when you're already full, it will also keep you naturally slim and healthy.

The secret of being slimmer and fitter is to get more pleasure from eating healthy food and from spending more time on physical activities that you really enjoy.

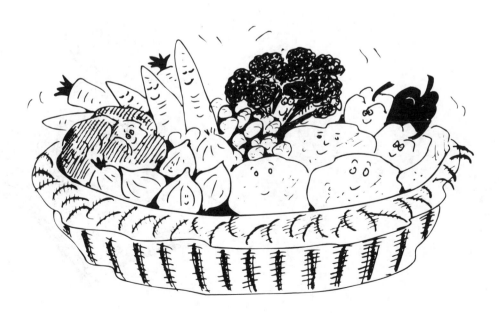

Food Diary 3

Time	Food and Drinks	Activity	Hunger Scale 1 2 3 4 5 6 7 8 9 10
9.00am	2 rashers bacon, 1 fried egg, beans, fried bread, 2 tomatoes, 2 sausages, toast, 2 mugs tea with sugar	Read paper.	8
2.30pm	Cheese and pickle sandwiches on white, 2 rounds, apple, Penguin, 2 cans Lilt	Driving.	5
4.30pm	2 mugs sweet tea, 3 digestives	Working.	4
6.30pm	Pizza, salad, fruit salad, 2 pints lager	None.	4
11.00pm	Double brandy, peanuts*	None.	6
*	Habits I could change?		

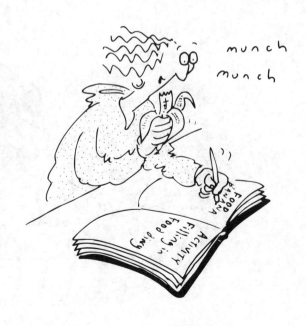

munch munch

Next Week's Diary

I expect you bought a big notebook for your **Food Diary** because it's about to become a bit more detailed. As well as noting what you eat, and when, include the following information as well:

- **How Hungry Were You, Exactly?**
  Many people I've worked with didn't know what it was like to get hungry. They were just seeing food and wanting it. A car that doesn't have oil flashes at you. Food is fuel, but you need to know where your indicators are. Get to know the signs of true physical hunger and note down in your diary where you are on the **Hunger Scale**.

- **What Else Were You Doing, Exactly?**
  Activities you associate with eating are important. Ideally there shouldn't be any. Eating's important enough to give it your full attention. After all, you wouldn't watch television while you were making love – would you? If you do – write it down.

Continue to look out for your eating patterns as you read through your diary.

Write down what happens when you run the *Think Before You Eat* strategy.

Take time to eat slowly and enjoy every mouthful.

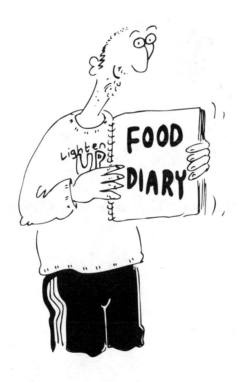

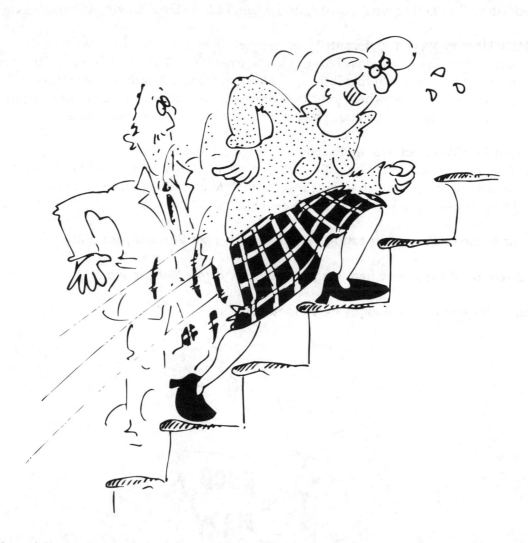

These folks have found the secret of being able to incorporate exercise into their lives.

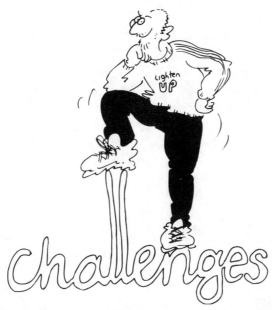

- Spend time everyday visualising yourself looking and feeling the way you would ideally like to be. The way you would look on Oscar Night if you'd been nominated for best actor/actress. Assume that you have a limitless budget and a couple of months to prepare. Remember – you get what you focus on.

- Make a habit of eating at least one meal a day without doing the crossword or running for the bus at the same time.

- Take an eating pattern that you want to change and change it now.

- Get yourself a **Fat Jar** and start filling it with **Fat-Burning Pills**: walk briskly for at least fifteen minutes every day.

- *Think Before You Eat*.

- Think about the pleasure you'll get from being slimmer, fitter and healthier and the pain you would experience if you failed to take control of your livelihood, and your health.

- Think about eating a healthier diet.

- Be aware of how food is making you feel.

- Concentrate on the taste.

- Over the next week, enjoy everything you eat and eat it slowly.

- At least twice a day, practise the **Open Door** exercise.

- Tell yourself a hundred times a day that you expect to be slimmer.

- Look at the recipes and try some of them out.

Week
What Gets You Going

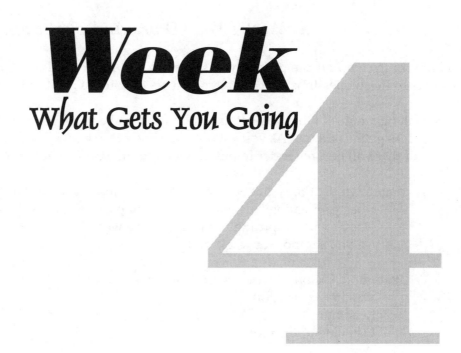

I'd spent the evening helping Lewis paint his kitchen. When we'd nearly finished I volunteered to fetch the takeaway and, while I waited for the order, I reached in my pocket for my wallet. It wasn't until I brought out a handful of scrunched up chocolate wrappers that I realised I'd taken the wrong jacket.

When we eventually sat down to eat, we were both tired and hungry. Nerves were frayed. Something to do with the smell of paint, maybe.

'Now that we've finished, I'm not sure I like this lime green,' said Lewis.

'You could have saved money by just papering it with Twix wrappers,' I suggested.

Lewis was defensive. 'I haven't worn that jacket in ages.'

'So how come there was a tube ticket with yesterday's on it amongst all the Twix papers? I thought you'd given up snacking all the time.'

'You try waiting on Vauxhall station when all the trains are running late. That platform's cold even in the middle of summer. One of those chocolate biscuits just tides me over until I get home. I don't have time to go to the café for a cup of tea, but there's a chocolate machine on the platform.'

'Well, I have to admit that's a reason.'

'It's not much of a reason though, is it?' he said. 'Not much of a reason for being twenty-eight pounds overweight.'

Last Week's Food Diary And Challenges

Did anything jump off the page at you last week? You may find it helpful to write down the answers to these questions. The more you write, the more you'll see.

❖ Making a note of what you eat at mealtimes soon becomes routine, though sometimes the snacks get missed out. As you get out your **Food Diary** each time, say to yourself: *'snacks?'* and that will be a reminder to put down anything you've had since the last meal.

❖ Writing down the times that you eat is easier if you keep your diary as you go along.
  – Does your eating cluster during certain parts of the day?
  – Does it vary according to the day of the week?
  – Do you eat more at weekends?

❖ What about the activities you associated with eating?
  – Watching television
  – Reading
  – Listening to the radio
  – Working
  – Driving
  – On the go

❖ How many meals did you manage to eat without doing anything else at the same time?

❖ What level are you at, typically, on the **Hunger Scale** before you eat?

❖ Were you aware that sometimes you might be eating when you were not really hungry?

❖ Did you change an eating pattern? How easy was it to do that?

❖ How was *Think Before You Eat*? Have you done it without planning to do it yet?

❖ How clear is your picture of yourself – the way you would *like* to be?

❖ How well did you get on with the **Open Door** exercise?

❖ What are you getting out of being more active?

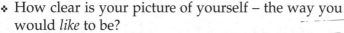

❖ How confident are you of your success?

❖ Is food making you feel good? Or is there still a bit of residual guilt around?

❖ How full is the **Fat Jar**?

How Are You Doing?

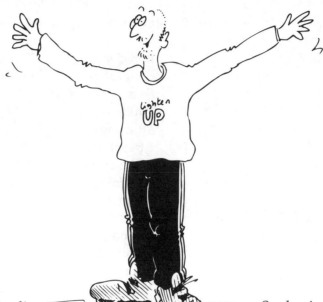

I know this sounds contradictory, but the **Food Diary** isn't about what you eat or what you're supposed to eat. I'm not asking you to write all this down so that you can criticise yourself. The reaction to what you write down should be, *'Hmm, that's interesting, there's a pattern there…I wonder why I do that? What else could I do?'* I don't want you to be weeping over the page or calling yourself names because you ate too many Jaffa Cakes. It doesn't matter. They're eaten.

The question I want you to ask yourself, if you notice that you seem to be putting rather a lot of ice cream into your Food Diary, is: *'What would be the most enjoyable way of turning this fat into fuel?'* Then go and do it. ASAP.

It's about being aware of what you do. There's a saying in management training:

'If you can't measure it, you can't manage it'.

It applies to eating just as well as it does to managing multi-billion-pound corporations.

So, having said all that, how *did* you get on with writing it all down last week? You were probably so busy with the diary that you didn't have much time to eat. Was it easy to make a regular note of what you ate? If not, what stopped you? Embarrassment often tops the list here, and if you can embarrass yourself, isn't it time to make a start on being a bit more frank? The other reason people give me for not keeping up with their Diary is that they couldn't be bothered.

My answer to that is, *'How much does being overweight bother you? What's it worth to make a change?'*

When you look through your entries for the week, I wonder if you find your eating patterns predictable, or surprising. Usually, you find some of both. I've asked a lot of questions on the left, but it's well worth taking the time to go through them slowly and think about the answers. They are important to you.

Feeling Fed up

Knowing what you need to eat to keep you healthy is all very well, but doing it is something else. In theory, realising you are hungry and that what you need is a banana, is pretty straightforward. In fact, popping out of the office for a minute because the pressure is getting to you and walking past the bakery just as they put the doughnuts in the window might be nearer to reality.

So, what are your triggers for overeating? If any of these get you going, tick them:

Parties	Boredom
Restaurants	Frustration
Eating alone	Fear
Eating with friends	Tiredness
Buffets	Mornings
Weddings	Afternoons
Diets	Being at work
Christmas	Holidays
Your birthday	Summer
Congratulating yourself	Winter
Comforting yourself	Insomnia
Loneliness	Feeling fat
Stress	Depression
Cooking	Anger

Of course, when you go to a restaurant or a party, it's great to enjoy the food. But if you eat twice as much as you need *just because* you're at your favourite Chinese – then it's going to make you feel bad. Which is a shame, because it should be an enjoyable experience. So, when you're triggered to overeat by any of the situations on this list, you're adding weight to the problem. You ate the bowl of cereal because you couldn't get to sleep and now you're going to wake up feeling fat and guilty.

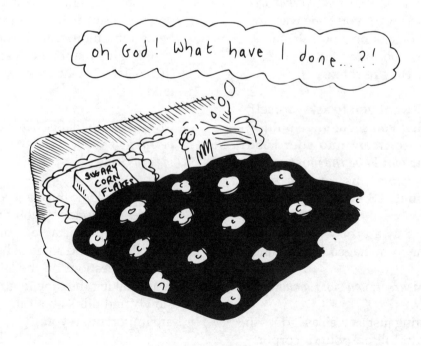

Eating Triggers

There are lots of reasons that trigger us to eat. The examples on the left are just some that people have given me over the years. Do any of them look familiar?

The more triggers you have to eat, the fatter you probably are. The key is learning to eat only when you are hungry and freeing yourself up to do something different when you are triggered to eat for other reasons.

Often, what triggers us to eat is that we want some pleasure. Many people associate pleasure with food. Or comfort, or reassurance, or support …

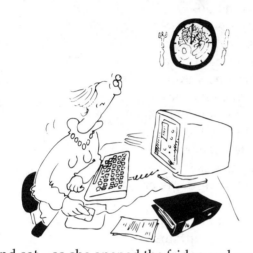

When you're upset, the first, most familiar suggestion your helpful subconscious mind comes up with is *'How about something salty, sugary or just plain fattening to cheer you up?'* Remember, you don't have to say yes to *everything* your subconscious suggests. You can politely ask it to come up with another alternative. Or, if it really isn't helpful, say something a little stronger. Like *'Shut up'*.

Mo used to come home from work to a flat that was often empty. She was tired, but she knew she had things to do, accounts, ironing, bill paying, phone calls. The easiest way to put it off was to sit down and eat – so she opened the fridge and grabbed whatever was sweet and easy and ready to hand. She always had a fridge full of stuff because, being in the catering business, she used to test recipes at home.

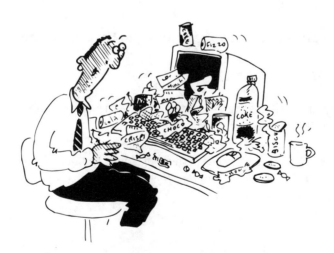

I remember one dreadful evening when she'd managed to get her VAT returns completed with the help of a sherry trifle. Ben and I turned up after a football match and she came to the kebab shop with us and ate more than her share! I had them both blaming me for that one. 'It's not my fault if you can't pass a kebab late at night,' I told Ben, 'and, as for you, Mo, why didn't you just say "no"? You've spent more time moaning about it than you spent on eating it in the first place.'

'I was trying to say "no" in my mind,' she said, 'but my body was already getting my purse and jacket'.

Displacement Activities

A good way to break the tyranny of your eating triggers is to learn to recognise them and then programme yourself to do something else instead – a **Displacement Activity.**

Go for a walk

Plan an outing on your next free day

Buy flowers for yourself or someone else

Buy a really nice wine and share it

See a movie

Go to an aerobics or stretch class

Go skating

Ride a bike

Picnic

Visit a bird sanctuary or aquarium

Take up knitting

Decorate a room

Mend something

Buy a tape or CD

Take music lessons

Have a massage

Phone a friend

Play cards with friends

Book a holiday

Go to a football game

Meditate

Start learning a language

Volunteer for a charity

Wash the leaves on your plants

Take a bath with a friend

Buy fancy underwear

Pick fresh fruit

Visit another town

Watch the sunset

Go swimming

Read a book

Window shop

Pet a cat or dog

Send a card

Start a new evening class

Go to a museum

Plant something

Listen to live music

Write a letter

Play tennis

Host a murder evening

Plan a party

Clear out a cupboard

Wash the curtains

Buy a hypnotic tape

Plan a holiday

Join a political party

Draw or paint a picture

Write down, in your diary, three that you are going to try over the next week.

They don't have to be from the list.

Remember that theory about it taking twenty to thirty times for a new pattern or behaviour to become automatic? Don't give up too soon.

And, if you end up eating the Danish pastry instead of going to your French class, forget about it. It's done. Do it differently next time. But don't prolong the agony when you've had a little lapse – you're only reinforcing your fat image when you do that.

Do Something Else

Doing something other than eating when you're not hungry will make you slimmer because anything you eat when you're not hungry turns straight into fat.

If you have been using food for anything but hunger, you are probably eating more than your body really needs. The challenge for you now is to meet those un-hungry needs some other way. Don't leave yourself vulnerable, lonely or un-comforted. Do something else. A Displacement Activity.

If you are triggered to eat for any other reason than hunger, ask yourself:

- What do I really want?

- What can I do (other than eating) to make myself feel good?

Finding something different that hits the right spot may take a little time. And doing it might meet with some resistance at first – in your own mind and in other people's. We tend to be creatures of habit and comfort. When we find something that makes us feel better, we usually stop looking for other alternatives, even if our chosen method (like eating) has negative side effects. I'm asking you to keep looking.

Look past the initial resistance, look past the first hurdles and see what your new patterns will do for you in future. Keep your eye on that and there's a good chance that you will start to enjoy doing things differently.

When an emotion creeps over you that used to trigger you to eat, you'll find yourself doing something else instead. And the more often you repeat your new behaviour, the easier it will become. Eventually you'll find your new habit has a stronger pull on you than eating used to have.

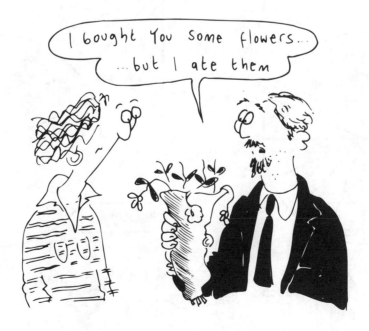

The Food Cake

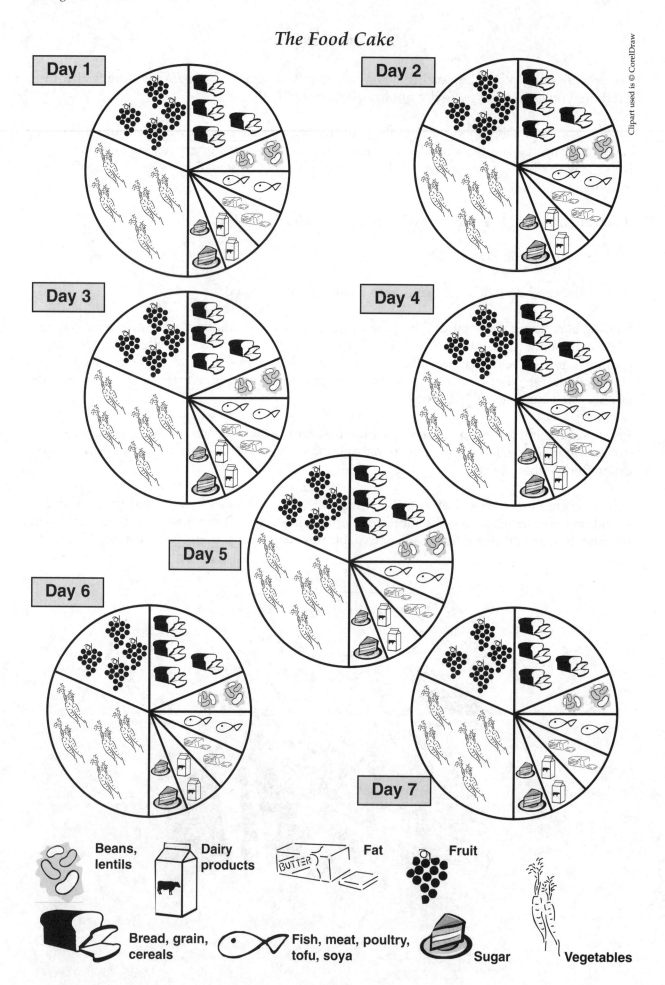

Day 1

Day 2

Day 3

Day 4

Day 5

Day 6

Day 7

Beans, lentils

Dairy products

Fat

Fruit

Bread, grain, cereals

Fish, meat, poultry, tofu, soya

Sugar

Vegetables

Clipart used is © CorelDraw

Introducing The Food Cake

This isn't a diet sheet, it's a way of showing you how healthy your diet is.

Food is Good For You

Food isn't the enemy. We need the right amount of the right food to make our bodies function at all. It's energy, it's fuel, it's essential. Not eating is always fatal, and starvation and malnutrition kill at least as many people as overeating and unbalanced eating.

The Food Cake

The **Food Cake** is your eating reference for the next five weeks. And that's all it is, a reference, *not* a set of rules.

It's not a strict regime or a complicated formula, it's just a simple, visual way of seeing whether you are eating a healthy, balanced selection of food every day.

You don't know in advance just how much slimmer you will become during that time. But, by looking at the **Food Cake** to see how much variety you have in your diet, you can steadily lose weight, while, at the same time ensuring that you are eating a good balance of foods from different food groups. Many diets cut out certain foods altogether but the **Food Cake** works on the principle that you need a little of everything and that too much of anything will turn to fat – even if it starts out as skinned chicken breasts and steamed spinach.

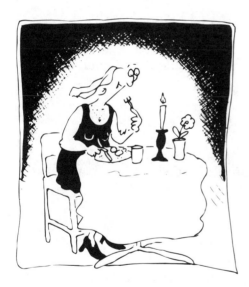

Guidelines

We based the **Food Cake** on the dietary guidelines developed by the U.S. Department of Agriculture and the Department of Health. They are guidelines for a balanced diet which includes a variety of foods from different food groups. This will help you to get the energy, protein, vitamins, minerals, and fibre you need for good health.

To make the cake easier to eat, the four food groups have been split into eight:

- Vegetables

- Fruits

- Cereals, grains and bread

- Beans and lentils

- Meat, fish, poultry, soya or tofu

- Dairy products

- Fats

- Sugar

Good Eating Guidelines:

- Eat as many fresh and natural products as possible, unrefined flour and grains.

- Cut out as many pre-packaged foods as possible.

- Drink plenty of fresh water.

- Limit your intake of red meat and include other sources of protein.

- Boil, steam or grill your food rather than frying it.

- Limit the use of oil.

- Cut down on sugary and fatty foods like cake, biscuits, crisps and sweets.

You will notice that I've included soya and the soya product tofu with meat and fish, rather than with the other beans and the lentils. This is simply because tofu is almost entirely protein and from a practical point of view it fits better into the meat and fish category.

Not Rules

Pleasure and Pain

A lifetime of food denial punctuated by occasional binges is a miserable way to live but it does serve the need for self-punishment that a lot of us seem to have. Most people on diets aim to cut out the binges – eventually. But of course, they can't, because a body can only take so much pain.

Some diets actually use this principle to their advantage by offering you a system which lets you binge on some food groups while cutting out others altogether. This provides pleasure and pain at the same time. However much cabbage soup or red wine or grapefruit you're allowed, you're bound to yearn for the scrambled eggs and bananas you're not supposed to eat. Diets like this are bound to be unbalanced and they often cause deficiencies in certain vital nutrients. A happy balance is the key to healthy eating, but you have to start being nice to yourself if you're going to achieve it.

Just make some copies of the **Food Cake** sheet in this chapter and each time you eat a serving from one of the above groups, colour it in. By the end of the day or week you will have a clearer picture of how varied your eating habits are and whether you are missing out on some foods and overloading on others.

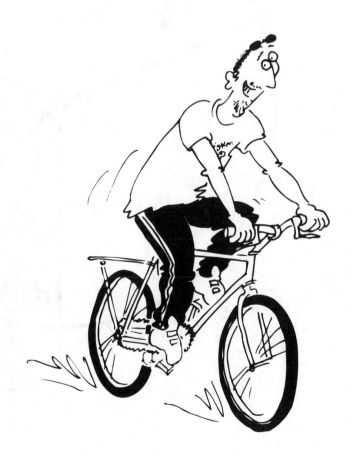

Lisa's Food Cake

- Bowl of unsweetened muesli with a handful of raisins
- Semi-skimmed milk
- Black coffee

- Tuna sandwich with salad
- 1 apple
- 2 pears
- 1 orange

- 3 cups of tea
- 2 litres water
- Black coffee

- Banoffee pie (2 large slices)

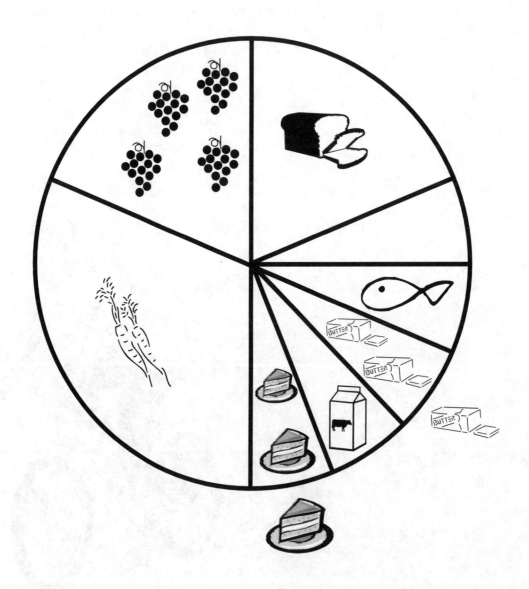

Clipart used is © CorelDraw

What's A Serving?

Each symbol on the **Food Cake** represents a serving of a particular food group.

Vegetables, beans or lentils   1 cup* of cooked vegetables

Fruit   1 large fruit (apple, orange, peach)
¼ cup of fresh juice
1 cup of berries or pineapple
2 handfuls of cherries or grapes
2 handfuls of raisins

Cereals, grains and bread   1 cup of cooked grain, such as rice, pasta, potatoes
1 cup of unsweetened cereal
2 slices of bread or 2 small rolls

Meat, poultry, fish, soya, tofu   3oz lean meat, poultry, fish, soya or tofu

Dairy foods   1 egg
2oz low fat cheese
1 cup non-fat milk, ½ cup semi-skimmed milk
½ cup low fat yoghurt

Fat   1 tablespoon of oil, margarine, butter
4 tablespoons of cream
Small handful of mixed nuts
Small handful of unsalted peanuts
Small handful of nuts and seeds
4 teaspoons of peanut butter
Small bag of crisps
Small portion of chips
A couple of biscuits

Sugar   1 tablespoon of sugar, honey or jam

* A cup is either a small tea or coffee cup or American measuring cup filled flat, not heaped.

More About The Cake

- If you choose high fat meat or poultry instead of lean, simply lose one of your daily allowances of fat. This means that all your fat may come from meat alone on that particular day. I wouldn't recommend this on a regular basis as meat is saturated fat, which should be limited. Your fat intake could come from other sources.

- You can do the same thing if you eat full fat instead of low fat dairy produce. Just count it as two fat servings instead of one. And, again, it's not a good idea to take all of your daily fat from dairy produce, because, like meat, it's saturated fat. *Remember*, variety is the key to balance and health.

- If you eat anything containing fat *and* sugar together, such as chocolate, cakes and biscuits, it's highly likely that you will consume or even exceed your fat and sugar servings in one go. If you work on the premise that four small biscuits contain all your fat and sugar for the day, then you'll start to get a clearer picture.

- Did you know that one Mars bar contains eight teaspoons of sugar? So be smart with cakes, biscuits and confectionery. If you fancy a little, have a little, but make sure the rest of your food that day contains no added fat or sugar.

- Vegetarians can substitute beans, lentils, tofu or soya for meat servings.

- If you don't like beans and lentils then substitute fish or poultry instead. It's a good idea to consume as many types of protein as possible.

- Avoid processed, ready-made meals if you can. They can be loaded with hidden fats and are often low in nutrients.

- Beware of low fat 'diet' products. They are often higher in sugar than their 'normal' alternatives and they are usually full of chemicals.

- Eat unrefined grains, cereals and breads, such as wholemeal bread, brown rice and pasta. They are higher in nutrients than refined produce.

- Add as many herbs and spices to your cooking as you like. They are full of goodness and add loads of flavour.

- Look to drink eight glasses of water a day and a minimum of four.

The greater variety of foods you include in your diet the healthier you will be.

How Much Is Enough?

Large, medium and small people can all use the same **Food Cake**. Servings of protein, fat, dairy products and sugar stay roughly the same for everyone. If you are a large (tall, not wide), or very active person, and you know you're registering high on the **Hunger Scale**, then help yourself to extra vegetables, fruit, cereals, grains and bread and any good sources of protein.

Daily Servings:

6 servings of vegetables
4 servings of fruit
4 servings of cereals, grains & bread
2 servings of beans and lentils
2 servings of meat, fish, poultry, soya or tofu
2 servings of dairy products
2 servings of fat
2 servings of sugar

How much you eat depends on how much your body needs. The only way to know this is to get to know yourself and that's what a lot of the exercises (the **Hunger Scale**, *Think Before You Eat* and the **Food Diary**) are all about. But, until you get to know yourself really well again (yes, you did know all this once, you've just forgotten), you can use the **Food Cake**.

Don't try to get it exactly right. It can be very difficult to work out exactly how much of everything you should eat, so I don't bother and I don't think it's necessary to be that precise. *But, most diets do, because a lot of people like that approach. It's easier to be told exactly what to do.* Unfortunately, it doesn't work when you put the book down and go off the diet. The **Food Cake** is a guide to what types of food you should be eating but only *you* will know how much. And you will know by listening to your body so you can eat when you're hungry and stop when you're full.

You can waste a lot of time weighing out rolled oats and counting beans. If you really must have a ritual, make it *Think Before You Eat*, not Weights and Measures. And if you've still got time on your hands and food on your mind, try the **What Do You Want?** exercises, either alone, or with a friend. Start getting to know the slimmer, happier You. Practise your **Daydreaming With Intent** until you have a bright, clear, compelling image of how you could look and be. You'll soon find it quite difficult to eat the kind of food your body doesn't need at times when it's not really hungry.

If you're smaller, or less active, or there are days when you don't feel very hungry, then you can eat less. You don't *have* to fill in every sector every day

Give Yourself Some Credit

- Whenever you score a hit in the **Food Diary,** for enjoying a meal, knowing when you're hungry or going for a walk instead of downing the seventh pint, congratulate yourself.

- Do your daydreaming practice at regular intervals. See yourself doing good things and taking recognition for them gracefully.

- Give yourself a pat on the back whenever you catch yourself doing something right and the **Food Diary** isn't at hand.

- Give yourself positive messages now and again.

- If you recognise the good things that happen and constantly look out for them, more and more good things will tend to happen.

Take responsibility for tracking your own triumphs. And remember, this is one situation where size really doesn't matter.

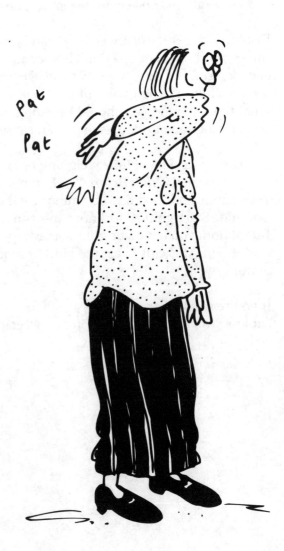

Recognition

I saw Mo at a wedding the other day. When the cake came round Mo waved the plate away and when I turned around from taking a piece for myself she was grinning like the Cheshire cat.

'What? What's funny? And why didn't you have any cake?' I asked her. 'Is it because you didn't make it and you don't think it's up to standard?'

'No, it's not that at all. I really didn't want any – and now, when I say "no" to something I don't want, I feel so pleased with myself, I'm kind of cheering in my head at my own achievement. And that makes me feel even better.'

It didn't even occur to me to laugh at her for congratulating herself over a piece of cake. How could I? – after the time we'd been through a few years ago when her weight seemed to be the only thing in her life she couldn't control and the one thing she cared about more than anything. I wish more people would give themselves that kind of credit. Congratulating yourself is the best way I know of making good behaviour stick, yet most people rely on others to tell them when they're doing well.

Successful people are different. *They are much better at recognising their own achievements. This is a really easy behaviour pattern to acquire.*

We live in a society which focuses on problems and the possibility of things going wrong. We are programmed to expect failure and we often don't even notice when we do get something right. In future, instead of re-living every defeat and disaster, make a mental note of every time you do something right, or even write it in the Diary. Keep it handy for an action replay when you need a boost.

Exercise In Comfort

Eat sensibly and take plenty of exercise.

Is that really all there is to becoming slimmer? Hardly a revelation you might think. But, if it's so easy, why do 95% of dieters still fail? We'll get on to that later. But for now, having talked about food, we have to take a look at the other side of the equation – how you burn it up once you've eaten it.

The Borg Scale works on the same principle as the **Hunger Scale**. And, like the **Hunger Scale**, most people react to it the first time by saying, *'Yes, but how do I know whether I'm at 6 or 7?'* And I say, *'Just behave as if you do know.'* And they go away and do it.

The Borg Scale

How hard am I working?

1	2	3	4	5	**6**	**7**	**8**	9	10

| Standing still | | | Gentle exercise
Breathing
   normally | | Comfortable exercise
Deep breathing
Really feel your body
   working
Burning fat | | | Out of breath
Really hard work
Not enjoying it
Burning sugar | |

When you are doing your continuous comfortable exercise, ask yourself, 'At what level am I working?' Grade it between 1 – 10.

You want to be between 6 – 7 – 8 for a period of fifteen minutes to one hour. Make sure it's comfortable and continuous. If you're out of breath, you may be working too hard.

Dieting doesn't change your body chemistry for the better, but being more active can. If you diet drastically your body will slow down and hoard more fat. But, if you become more active, you will adjust your personal thermostat so that you burn more fuel.

Dieting alone creates confusion and the body will resist using fat. Use the Borg Scale to make sure you are working at the right level.

Move It And Lose It

There are as many mixed messages about exercise as there are about diet. It's a bit like the veggie versus carnivore battle. It's hard to convince a dedicated couch potato that his neighbour is really cycling to work by choice. And the jogger, dependent on his daily endorphin high, pities the flabby commuter gasping for breath as he heaves himself onto the train at the last minute.

So, who's right?

There are undoubtedly some troubled souls who exercise beyond all need or capacity. Either they don't have much of a home life or they really enjoy that ultrasound machine that the sports physios tape you up to when you've injured your leg yet again. But the people who love to move and exercise their bodies have too much respect for themselves to risk injury and they know that if it hurts it's not doing them any good.

But how do you reassure the thousands of people who are already totally convinced that exercise is going to hurt? They know that the only reason for doing it is to burn as many calories as fast as possible and get it over with. The idea of enjoying it for it's own sake is incomprehensible to them.

Make these your exercise goals:

- **To teach your body to burn fat**

- **To feel good for no good reason**

- **To have fun**

Fat is the energy source we use while we're sleeping, sitting, working and even eating. Fit people are efficient at using it and fat people are efficient at storing it.

In order for the body to burn fat, it needs a large amount of oxygen. However, if you are out of breath when you exercise, you won't be getting enough oxygen and your body will be working too hard. Remember, the body needs oxygen to burn fat. If you're working too hard and you're out of breath you will be burning more sugar than fat.

When you exercise, enjoy the process. Expect to feel those endolphins* swimming around your body and making you feel good.

*I may be dyslexic, but I do know how to spell endorphins. I just think endolphins sound like more fun.

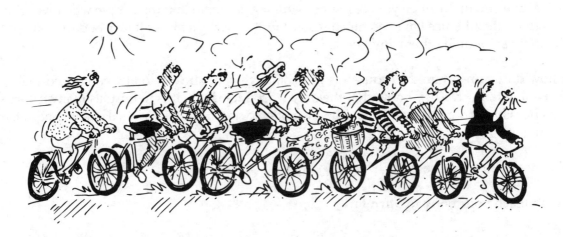

It's how you get there,
and the company you keep
that determines the shape
you're in when you arrive

Sasha Moran

The Cure For Fat

Being fat tends to make you even fatter. Fatness is a vicious circle because body chemistry favours stability. Fat people tend to take less exercise than thin ones because it's harder for them. So they don't build up their muscles in the same way and it's muscle that burns fat. So, when muscle gives way to fat through inactivity, you burn less of that fat when you do exercise. As if that wasn't bad enough, the chemistry of the remaining muscle changes in such a way as to require fewer calories.

Inactivity is definitely the most important factor in gaining weight. But drastic dieting doesn't help. A lot of overweight people prefer to diet rather than exercise but the problem then is that your body will react to a sudden reduction in food by slowing down your metabolism. After dieting for two weeks, your metabolic rate can drop by 20%. That's the *bad news*.

The *good news* is that exercise can increase your metabolic rate, and not just when you're exercising.

The main function of fat is to be used for energy by the muscles. A lot of diet systems suggest that it's hard to burn fat but that's not actually true. We burn fat all the time. 70% of our muscles' energy needs come from fat and the main benefit of exercise is to burn it.

Burning calories is another benefit, but it tends to be over-emphasised because what people often forget is that they are burning calories all the time, even when they're asleep. You might only burn a couple of biscuits worth in an exercise session but that doesn't matter. What really matters is that the more exercise you do the more your metabolism speeds up. Not only do you digest food quicker, you are also building up your lean muscle which uses more calories. This takes time. If you want to change something as fundamental as your body chemistry, it's a good idea to do it at a pace which suits your body. That might mean telling your mind to be patient. It helps if, while you are waiting, you bear in mind that every time you walk up the escalator or leave the car in the garage, you are turning up your internal thermostat and burning more fuel.

Exercise is the fountain of youth. The main reason why people tend to put on weight as they get older is that they exercise less. Their muscles become less dense, less lean and more fatty. Children are almost never still. That's why they're so tiring to live with and also why they are usually thinner than grown-ups. They're burning calories as quickly as they eat them. Unfortunately, as more children spend their leisure time sitting in front of a screen rather than playing their own games, more and more of them are becoming as overweight as their parents.

Adults (and overweight children) can reverse the fat trend simply by taking more exercise.

If you have been inactive for some time, please consult your doctor before starting an exercise routine or increasing your activity levels.

Outcomes...

Outcomes are like destinations. You have to decide on them in advance if you want to get anywhere. Having a destination in mind is of primary importance in your journey to becoming slimmer, fitter, healthier.

- Today I am going to eat along the lines of the categories on the Food Cake.

- Today I am going to eat only when I'm more than 7 on the Hunger Scale.

- Today I am going to cycle to work and walk up the escalators.

- Today I am going to work out for twenty minutes and put five pence in the *Fat Jar* as well.

- Today I am going to give myself credit every time I do something positive.

- Today I am going to spend five minutes visualising myself being even slimmer, fitter and healthier.

- Today I am going to feel good and release any stress.

When you get into the habit of setting and achieving your **Outcomes**, you are quite likely to turn into a success junkie. You'll want to keep achieving and succeeding. The buzz you'll get from repeatedly reaching the goals you set yourself will create its own momentum.

If you don't get your Outcome, find out why, learn from it and do something different next time.

...Are Like Destinations

If you already have an **Outcome** for this programme, how about setting **Outcomes** for what you do on a daily, weekly or monthly basis? It could be as simple as following the weekly **Challenges** on a daily basis.

By setting and achieving **Outcomes**, you will get into the habit of experiencing success. If you want to get more out of your daily life, start setting yourself **Outcomes** for whatever you do.

For example, if you are going out with some friends, ask yourself, *'What do I want from this evening?'* If you were to set yourself an **Outcome** like: *'I'm going to have a good time and enjoy myself,'* then that's what you are going to get. You get what you focus on.

Another example would be to ask yourself, *'What do I want to get out of today?'* You might set yourself an **Outcome** like: *'Eating three sensible meals, taking my FAT-burning pill and having some fun.'* If you commit to doing this, then that's what you are going to get.

- What do you want to achieve this time tomorrow?

- What do you want to achieve this time next week?

Think of the feelings you get when you accomplish something. Even the feeling you get when you tick an item off your "To Do" list. It doesn't matter whether it's cleaning the fridge out or completing your first novel. You'll get that same good feeling when you achieve your **Outcomes** and feel the satisfaction of taking positive action that is making you slimmer, fitter and healthier.

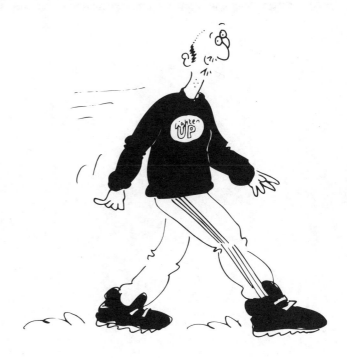

Food Diary 4

Time	Food and Drinks	Activity	Hunger Scale 1 2 3 4 5 6 7 8 9 10
7.00am	2 black coffees, ½ grapefruit	Making children's breakfast. Feeling tired.	4
10.00am	2 mugs of tea, Kit Kat	Working. Couldn't concentrate.	5
12.30pm	Piece of flapjack, apple, 2 oranges, packet crisps	Working. Very. stressed.	8
5.30pm	2 fish fingers, orange, Diet Coke	Feeding children.	5
9.00pm	Pizza and salad, 2 glasses wine	Nothing. Feeling relaxed.	7

1 litre water during day
3 "fat-burning pills"

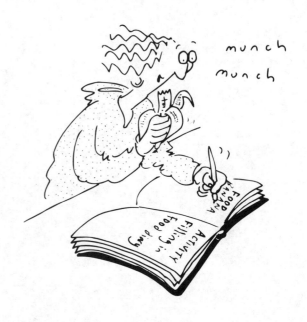

munch munch

Next Week's Diary

Your Food Diary will be looking rather well-used by now, you probably have a few food splodges on it and it's looking a bit dog-eared. That's great. Keep going.

- Did you know that the best way to store food is to eat it? Even freezer foods have an eat-by date. But once it's inside you, your body will obligingly store as much food as you like in the form of fat and it will keep indefinitely. It's an efficient system if you live in a cave without supermarkets or refrigeration.

- Continue to write down what you're eating and make a note of any activities associated with eating.

- Take some copies of the **Food Cake**. Enough for the next week, or fortnight. Or seven times the number of chapters left in the book. Or maybe enough to last until the millennium. Depending on how pessimistic or optimistic you are.

- Colour in the foods you eat every day. You can't carry foods forward to the next day, or spread one day's virtuous eating over a whole week. If you eat enough spinach for seven days on Monday, you'll just be wasting it. There won't be enough room to fill it in on Monday's cake and your body isn't going to get more than one day's benefit from it either.

- If you eat *more* of anything than your daily allowance, just draw it in at the side and colour it. It still counts.

- Write down what triggered you to eat – hunger, boredom, etc.

- Don't forget to log your exercise.

- Notice any feelings associated with food. How food makes you feel, or, perhaps, what makes you feel like food.

- Use the **Hunger Scale**. If you ask yourself how hungry you are and the answer is less than 5, the chances are you're not really hungry. In that case, look to do something else instead.

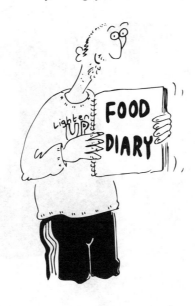

If *you* are ⌐triggered to eat,⌐ do something else instead.
And feel good – *you deserve it.*

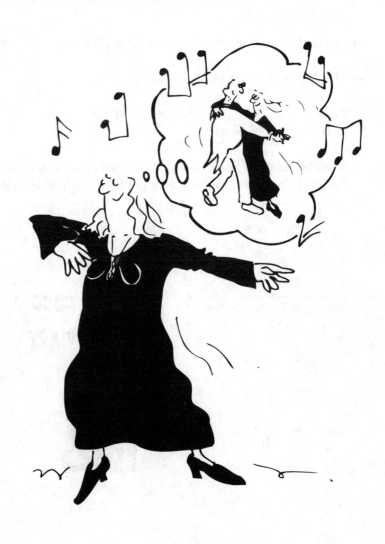

➠ Do all the exercises for this week.

➠ Continue to use the *Think Before You Eat* strategy.

➠ Eat when you are registering above 5 on your **Hunger Scale**.

➠ If you think about eating when you are at less than 5, substitute another activity, like reading a book or going for a walk. Find other ways of feeling good.

➠ Keep filling your **Fat Jar** with **Fat-Burning Pills** – walk briskly for at least fifteen minutes a day, but take more exercise if you feel you can.

➠ Separate eating from other activities.

➠ Give yourself credit for your actions.

➠ Set yourself daily **Outcomes**.

➠ Continue with the **Open Door** exercise. The more you see, hear and feel yourself being slimmer, the more quickly you'll achieve it.

➠ Do something different when you are triggered to eat for reasons other than hunger. Take up some **Displacement Activities** and feel good for no good reason.

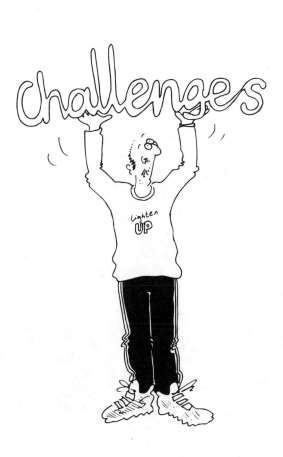

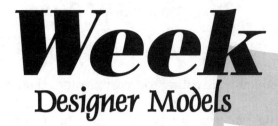

Week
Designer Models

When I introduced my first slimming group to the **Food Cake** they really liked it because it looked more like rules which was what they were used to when they went on a diet.

'It's not rules,' I told them, 'it's guidelines'.

'Same difference,' said Ben. And the others agreed with him.

After a stressful day at work I stopped by Lisa and Mo's flat, kind of hoping I might persuade one of them to try out the new Thai restaurant with me. Lisa opened the door and I followed her in but she turned down my invitation straight away.

'Why? Have you eaten already?' I asked her.

'Sort of. You know that **Food Cake**?' she produced her piece of paper, with her choices filled in.

It looked pretty good. 'That's a lot of fruit by your standards,' I remarked.

'I know, I used to think fruit was too messy to bother with at work. It was easier to have a biscuit. But watch this, I haven't finished filling it in.' She got a marker and filled in a slice of cake, then added another one outside the circle.

I just looked at her. 'Was that dinner?'

'It wasn't meant to be. I'd been brilliant all day, because I thought I was going to the cinema tonight with Lewis. When I got home there was a message on the answering machine saying he's been sent up to Sunderland on a project for a few days.' She caught sight of my face – I can never get my expression organised fast enough. 'OK, I know a trip to the pictures is no big deal, but it was just the change of plan. I felt kind of flat. So I got the banoffee pie out of the freezer and had a slice. Then I had another one. Now I feel flat *and* fat.'

Lisa and I compromised and went to see the film instead of going out to dinner. But I could tell the banoffee pie was weighing heavily on her mind. 'Rules are rules,' she said, over a coffee, later on.

'Rules are meant to be broken,' I told her. 'That's why the **Food Cake** isn't a rule. Rules restrict you. Eating triggers are like rules you made for yourself and I want you to break them. You didn't *have* to eat junk food just because you were disappointed, did you?'

Last Week's Food Diary

❖ How many **Fat-Burning Pills** did you take and put in your **Fat Jar**?

❖ Did you notice when you were eating for reasons other than hunger?

❖ Which of your eating patterns did you change; was it a time-linked or a food-linked activity?

❖ How many times did you eat without doing anything else at the same time?

❖ Did you run the **Open Door** exercise? What did you see and hear when you'd achieved the size and shape you wanted to be?

❖ If *Think Before You Eat* becomes a reflex reaction now, what else might change?

❖ How do you feel about filling in the **Food Cake**? Are you learning anything from that exercise?

❖ Are you displacing any of your snacks with other activities?

❖ How often do you give yourself credit for your achievements, large or small?

❖ What about the **Outcomes** you are setting? Are they working out? And are you setting up ones you really *want* to aim for – or ones you think you *ought* to aim for?

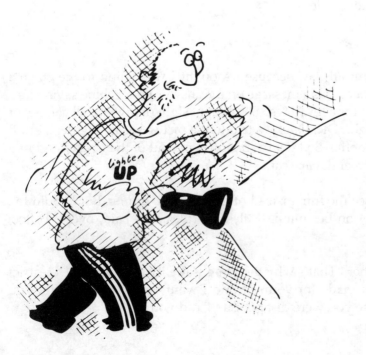

How Are You Doing?

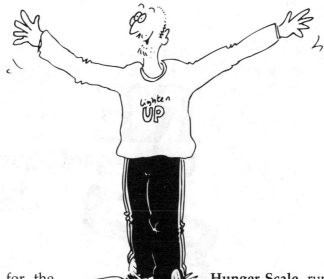

Lightening Up strikes for the fifth week, and you are now more than halfway through the course. You are probably noticing that you are taking more exercise than you've been used to. And you can imagine how it will feel to be even more active by next week. Did you make a note of *all* your regular exercise; running up stairs, cycling to work, walking to the shops?

I am pretty sure you're enjoying the experience of eating when you're not doing anything else at the same time. Is it getting easier? And when you do manage to concentrate on eating, how does the food taste? Are you eating more or less this way?

What about the feelings that might have been making you eat when you weren't really hungry? Have you discovered whether you eat when you're depressed? Happy? Anxious? Angry? Lonely? If you find yourself eating at less than five on the **Hunger Scale**, run a quick check for the presence of one of those emotions – or whichever feelings make you fall into the comfort eating trap.

Of the changes you made last week, which was the easiest? Was there something that fell into place so naturally that you wondered why you never did it before? And were there any that you really had to struggle with? What changes do *you* wish you had made last week that you think you could make over the next week?

What surprised you most about last week? *It may not be directly to do with eating.*

This is a good time to think back over the past four weeks and really take notice of all your positive actions. Congratulate yourself. It's also a good idea to renew your desire and commitment to becoming slimmer, fitter and healthier.

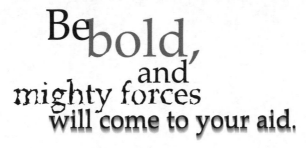

Be bold, and mighty forces will come to your aid.

REtakes are no problem – you have an *unlimited* time budget

If you want to double double your success rate, you may have to double double your failure rate first.

Lapsing, Relapsing And Collapsing

I want you to be able to distinguish between a **Lapse,** a **Relapse** and a total **Collapse.**

Lapses and Relapses are nothing to worry about. They are just behaviour patterns.

Collapses are more serious because they are based on beliefs, not behaviour.

A Lapse is a slight error or slip, the instance of backsliding. It is a discrete event, like eating crisps and peanuts all night at a party, or a whole tub of ice cream one lonely evening at home, or getting up too late to walk to work for a few days. It doesn't matter. Once it's done (or not done) it's over with.

This is when you have the unique opportunity to learn. You don't need to make the same mistake again.

A Relapse is when you manage to string a whole series of lapses together so that it starts to look like the state you were in before you started changing.

Even in this situation you have the capability to change things. Remember it's up to you, no one else is involved. It takes only a second to change. Be willing to do whatever it takes to get your **Outcome.**

A Collapse happens when you start believing again your old negative beliefs about yourself. It happens when you feel like it's not worth bothering to change any more or when you find you get just as much satisfaction from whining about your weight as you would from being slim.

This is the time to reflect on what happened. But, don't pause for long. You can soon be ready to turn things around and start again, with the benefit of hindsight. You can use the Success formula on the next page to turn all your perceived failures into successes.

Now move on.

The Success Formula

Success Is On The Other Side Of Failure

Step One   Notice yourself:

- making a mistake.

- talking to yourself in a self-defeating way.

- giving yourself a hard time.

Step Two   STOP. Pause and halt the process for a moment.

Step Three   Talk to yourself constructively, encouragingly.

Step Four   Become curious about what made you behave the way you did. Laugh at it. The behaviour isn't important. Your response to it is what matters.

Step Five   Ask yourself some useful questions: 'What specifically triggered me to behave this way? What started the overeating or the chocolate binge? What was I thinking about just before I did it?

Step Six   When you understand why you did what you did, ask yourself: *'What will I do differently next time it happens, so that I get a different* **Outcome** *– one that doesn't involve eating?'*

Step Seven   Consider the alternative courses of action:

- go for a walk.

- telephone a friend.

- have a bath.

Step Eight   Come up with your own strategy: if you don't learn from your mistakes, you'll carry them with you and make them again.

Step Nine   Look, learn and move on.

No Such Thing As Failure

The single **stupidest**

sentence ever in the

history of the

English language

is: '**Do it right the first time.'**
Nobody ever did anything even
half-interesting right the *41st* time.
Tom Peters

Edison was given the finance to make an electric light bulb, an idea which had been the despair of inventors for fifty years. It took him fourteen months of trial and error to find a suitable filament and he got it wrong hundreds of times before he got it right. But every time he tried an unsuitable material he merely took the view that he had eliminated another possibility and was one step closer to finding a permanent solution to the challenge.

There is an old saying that *'a path with no obstacles goes nowhere'*. There are going to be times when you make a mistake or think you've failed. Most of us fear failure because we think it means that we *are* failures. But failure is just something you have to do. It's always on the other side of success. When we get things wrong, it's an ideal opportunity to learn.

What you do is less important than your response to what you do.

So if you get stressed and you overeat, or you're tired or bored and you overeat, just say *'OK, that's what I did this time – what will I do differently next time?'*

Think about how you learned to drive or ride a bike. You probably didn't get it right first time. The mistakes you made were signposts that gave you the opportunity to learn.

Dieters are always one mouthful away from failure. One piece of chocolate or a late night binge and they think, *'I've blown it.'*

What a great excuse to dive back into the old bad habits!

The successful slimmers I've worked with have used experiences like this as opportunities to learn. Keep learning. Use the **Success Formula** on the left hand side to help you.

Drinking Water

- Drink a glass of water in the morning before breakfast.

- Accompany hot drinks with a glass of hot water.

- When you drink alcohol, wherever possible drink water as well.

- In cold weather drink warmer water.

- Take water with you on long car journeys or to work.

- Drink little and often. You will be surprised at how much water you can drink.

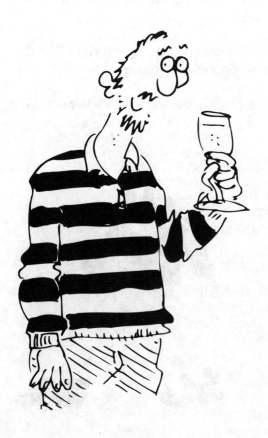

A Well Of Information

Drink lots of water

Two to three litres a day, preferably pure, although everything you drink is water based: orange juice, squash, even cola, coffee and tea. But the more things that are added to it, the longer it will take to extract the vital water. So if your favourite drinks are full of E numbers (chemicals) or caffeine (some soft drinks contain both) it won't be as beneficial to your system. Also, most soft drinks are full of sugar – between seven and fifteen spoonfuls!

Another thing to remember is that cola and similar drinks as well as coffee and tea, are diuretics, which means they actually dehydrate you by making you secrete more fluid than you take in. That could be another reason why some people just feel lousy a lot of the time. They're dehydrated.

The bottom line is that water in its purest form is how the body likes it.

WATER is an essential part of our bodily needs, second only to oxygen. It makes up approximately 55 – 65% of an adult's body weight and approximately 75% of a child's.

WATER: two litres are lost on average very twenty-four hours. This loss rises dramatically during exercise, depending on the duration and intensity of the exercise, your level of hydration before you start and the air temperature.

WATER loss accounts for the weight loss you measure immediately after exercise.

WATER is used by the body to aid temperature control; more is needed in hot weather. In situations where people sweat excessively, such as hot weather, exercise or illness, it's important to drink a lot more water.

WATER is essential to digestion and elimination. As a cleanser, it's crucial in allowing the kidneys to flush out toxins more effectively. Constant replenishment is vital to feeling and looking good.

WATER acts as a lubricant in the joints and between internal organs, keeping cells moist and allowing the passage of all manner of internal substances between cells and blood vessels.

...EVERYWHERE...

Fruit And Vegetables

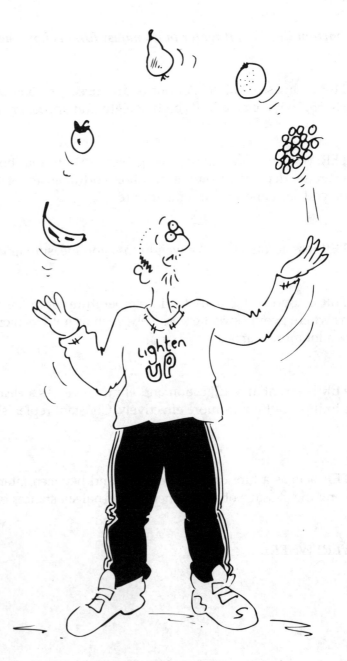

Fruit and veg are more fun than junk food.

Old Wives' Tales?

For many people, filling in the **Food Cake** highlights a lack of fruit and vegetables and gives them an incentive to include more fresh products in their daily food choices.

Carrots help you see in the dark* and broccoli makes your hair curl**? Maybe, maybe not. But the old message that people who eat their greens will grow up to be big strong boys (or girls) is true. The propaganda machine for vegetables started rolling during the Second World War when meat and sweets were rationed and expensive and the government was trying to put a positive spin on cabbage and turnips. It wasn't until later that the health services looked at their statistics and realised the hype had proved spectacularly true! During the years of rationing there was a marked fall in heart disease, high blood pressure and diabetes.

Opticians didn't go out of business and neither did hairdressers, although the pressure on a lot of GP's surgeries certainly eased. But right now, instead of a choice between a couple of apples or no pudding, we have fifty-two*** flavours of Ben & Jerry's. It might be a good idea to learn how to create our own healthy eating plan, because the government isn't going to do it for us.

Science is constantly researching the link between plenty of fresh, natural fruit and vegetables with good health. Recently the American Institute for cancer research estimates that as many as 40% of all cancers in men and 60% of those in women are linked to poor diet.

We are all natural, organic creatures. We are not made of additives, chemicals and preservatives. Our bodies naturally want fresh healthy fruit and vegetables to keep us full of health, energy and vitality.

* Yes
** No
*** Probably

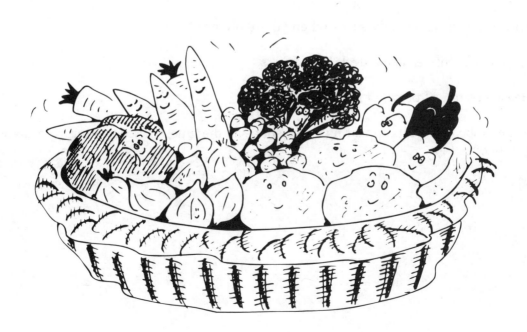

113

Fruit And Vegetables

One Food Cake serving is:

> **1 cup of raw vegetables**
> **1 large fruit**
> **¼ cup of fresh juice**
> **1 cup of berries or pineapple**
> **20 cherries or 20 grapes**
> **4 tablespoons of raisins**

Vegetables

Variety is the spice of life, and there's nothing to stop you adding herbs and spices to your vegetables and salads. With a little planning and creativity you can make them a particularly enjoyable, major part of your diet.

Make salads and vegetables a basic part of main meals.

Cook vegetables in different ways – steam or roast them to get a better flavour.

Frozen vegetables are better than no vegetables.

In restaurants the healthiest menu option is usually the one with most fresh vegetables.

Use fresh vegetables when you want a snack: celery or carrots for example.

Fruit

Fruit juices are good but make sure they are 100% pure wherever possible.

Add fruits to breakfast cereals.

Keep fruit available as a handy snack when you're hungry.

Make your own, unsweetened, fresh fruit drinks.

Eat at least a couple of pieces of fruit each day.

There seem to be new fruits appearing in the shops all the time, so, keep eating your favourites, but try new ones too.

Raw Energy

Vegetables

Vegetables should be a major part of a healthy, balanced diet. They are an excellent form of carbohydrate and contain lots of vitamins (lots of A and C) and minerals (iron and magnesium). They are a valuable source of antioxidants which help prevent against degenerative diseases, including cancer and heart disease. They contain soluble and insoluble fibre, which help to lower blood cholesterol levels. They are low in calories and fat and some of them are low in sugar too, so they are generally good news for people wanting to lose weight.

A lot of people don't eat many vegetables because they think they are boring and time consuming to prepare. That's not true. And you will find, by increasing your daily intake, that they start to taste much better as you now eat more of them in greater variety. They will also fill you up and help you become slimmer. Eat them whenever you're hungry.

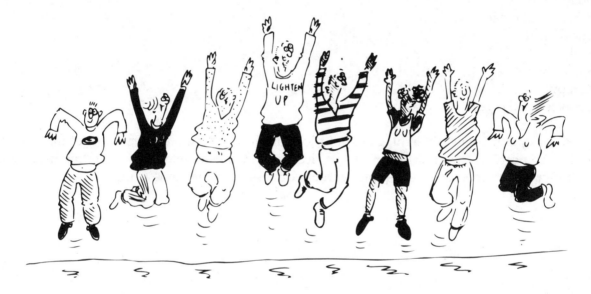

Fruit

Fruit plays an important part in a balanced diet. Many fruits contain lots of vitamins (particularly A and C), fibre and minerals. They are low in calories and fat and they are handy for snacks. Yes, they do contain sugar, but they aren't empty calories like candyfloss – they are so rich in so many other nutrients that they are well worth eating.

Bread, Cereals And Grains

One Food Cake Serving is: **1 cup of cooked grains, such as rice, pasta, potatoes**
                                        1 cup of unsweetened cereal
                                        2 slices of bread or 2 small rolls

Unrefined, whole products are the best, so, experiment with some that are new to you. Most of them only need boiling so they are simple to prepare although some of them take a little time.

All of these make a good base for a meal:

Rice, preferably brown
Pasta, preferably brown
Potatoes
Couscous
Bulgur wheat
Wholemeal bread
Buckwheat
Millet
Spelt
Keniou
Unsweetened cereals

If you fancy something different, go to your local health food shop and try some of the weirder grains. You can boil most of them just like rice – easy. Other vegetables – including beans and lentils – provide good quality, complex carbohydrates and so do some fruits.

High Quality Stodge

An easy way to change your body is to eat the highest quality, lowest fat and highest volume foods. These are complex carbohydrates which release energy over long time periods and stop you feeling hungry. They include bread, cereals, grains and potatoes, they taste starchy and they are high in nutritional value unless they've been processed or refined. Up to 25% of the calorific content can be burned up during digestion.

They should provide about 50% of our daily diet and it's a good idea to include at least one complex carbohydrate with each meal. Wherever possible, choose an unprocessed whole grain, or products made with unrefined flour and no added sugars or salt. These unprocessed foods are a good source of fibre and give you plenty of energy.

Processed foods, like white flour, white rice, normal pasta and most bread, have lost their tough seeds and fibres which help the gut deal with the food and which also contain some of the vitamins and minerals as well. These refined foods are much lower in both fibre and nutritional value.

There are three forms of carbohydrate: sugars, starch and fibre. Both fibre and starch are called complex carbohydrates and these foods are an essential part of a balanced healthy diet.

Unfortunately, it's sugars, or simple carbohydrates, in cakes, sweets, biscuits and soft drinks, which are a lot more tempting to most people. And not only are they full of sugar, some of them have a lot of hidden fat as well. These simple carbohydrates, or sugars, stimulate insulin release. Insulin is related to hunger so this is another reason why people who eat simple sugars feel hungry again faster than people who eat complex sugars.

Moving away from the simple sugars towards more complex carbohydrates and vegetables is a wise decision.

If you're stuck for ideas, use some of the recipes at the back of this book. Or go and buy one of the hundreds of easy and appealing cookery books with imaginative recipes for preparing grains.

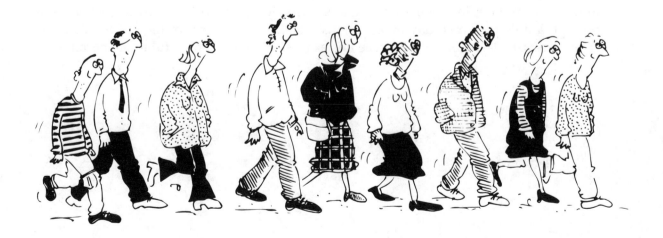

117

Changing Your Association With Food

Is there a dominant food you find particularly hard to resist? Chocolate, crisps, cola? If you feel you are developing a dependency relationship with this food, you can Change Your Association with it – forever if you want. Get someone to read this out to you and find a quiet comfortable place where you won't be disturbed for four or five minutes. It's not a good one to try on the tube home from work, or in the pub on a Saturday night.

- First close your eyes and take a couple of deep breaths.

- Think of the food that you would like to stop eating.

- Visualise this food in front of you. If you can taste it and smell it as soon as you picture it, then you have a strong association with it.

- Put this food image into a framed picture.

- Push the picture a few feet further away.

- If the picture is in colour, turn down the brightness so that it's dark, or black and white.

- Keep in mind this dull picture. Think of a smell you find disgusting. Breathe the smell deeply into your lungs. If it's not bad enough, find a worse one.

- With that smell in your nose, think now of a particular taste you find unpleasant or foul.

- Roll the taste round your mouth. You don't have to swallow.

- Keeping that foul taste in your mouth, bring back the dull picture.

- With the picture in front of you, surround it with the disgusting smell you conjured up.

- Take the food out of the picture and bring it towards you, smelling the obnoxious smell and tasting the revolting taste you added to it.

- Go on, treat yourself. Have a bite. Or would you rather not?

- In order to re-condition yourself for total success and permanent pleasure, put yourself through a little pain each day by consciously making the effort to think of this horrible smell and taste. The more you practise this exercise, the more powerful it will become.

Talking Back

When the crisps tell you to eat them, tell them to shut up.

Some people feel drawn towards eating sweet, fattening food. They feel almost compelled to eat them. Lisa used to sit at her desk battling with herself over whether or not to buy a bar of chocolate from the vending machine. The chocolate was talking to her, *'eat me, eat me now…'* and, more often than not, she did. Afterwards she usually wished she hadn't and she felt fat, full and sometimes guilty.

Way back at the beginning, I remember asking her how she saw herself and she said to me, *'I wish I could just scrape this lard off my thighs'*. Well, apart from the fact that she didn't have lardy thighs, not that I could see anyway, what an attractive picture that was! Not.

After that, I did the exercise on the left with her a couple of times and she was able to change her association with those chocolate bars. She got so that she felt quite negative about them. You may not want to do that if you love chocolate and you want to indulge occasionally, but it's worked for Lisa. In fact, only recently she told me that she's installed a new voice inside her head which asks her, *'Do you like it enough to wear it?'*

The way to stay slim is to reshuffle your positive and negative associations so that the exercise and healthy eating are easy and fun, and the slobbing and stuffing are painful and uncomfortable.

If you're forcing yourself into a lifestyle you hate, you'll never keep it up. Jerry Hall was once asked on a chat show how she kept slim. Did she have a punishing exercise routine? *'No,'* she said. *'It must be the shopping, all that running in and out of stores and trying on clothes. That bending and stretching really tones you up.'*

Use pleasure as your ally. And that includes conjuring up some compellingly attractive images of yourself and keeping them in mind.

Are there any particular sugary or fattening foods that you would like to cut out of your diet?

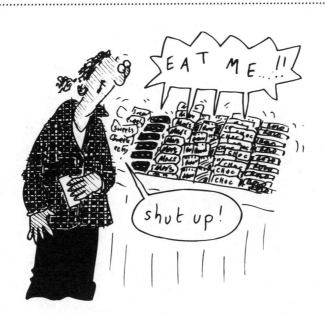

Think Before You Shop

How to tell when you're ready to go shopping:

- You have planned your meals for the next week.

- You have made a list.

- You have your magnifying glass to read the labels so you can reject the ones with too many chemicals.

- You're looking forward to buying some fresh foods and you don't mind putting in a bit of extra time on the preparation (check out some of the recipes at the back of the book).

- You have just had a meal.

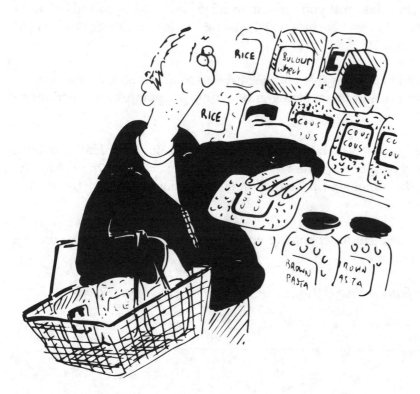

It's Tough Going Shopping

What's so hard about shopping? A trip to the superstore can be the fastest way to sabotage a weight-loss initiative. You need strength and determination to survive. And like most military operations, it needs precise planning if you are to succeed.

Preparing for a shopping trip takes skill and patience. I understand there's going to be an NVQ in shopping soon and that sounds like a great idea to me. It's definitely too technical for the inexperienced – I shared a house once with a guy who lived on takeaways. If you sent him out for the week's groceries – even with a list – he had no idea how to check for furry fruit at the bottom of a carton and he certainly couldn't tell the difference between fat free, sugar free, fruit free, and live or dead yoghurt.

Supermarkets, not surprisingly, are designed with the profit of the shareholders rather than health of the shoppers in mind. The good thing about them is that there is plenty of choice and the organic section seems to be getting larger all the time. The *Think Before You Eat* strategy applies to shopping as well and **Thinking Before You Shop** is something you can quickly train yourself (and sometimes even other members of your household) to do. Don't be too optimistic about this though, start on yourself.

Everybody knows that the big food stores are arranged to confuse you. As soon as you memorise a layout it gets changed so you'll end up looking at stuff you never planned to buy. Most people also realise that the fruit and veggies are at the beginning where your resistance to buying is higher (also they tend to get squashed by the beer you sling in at the end). Fresh produce is often a lower profit margin item because of its short shelf life.

There are bright, sugary fattening foods at the checkout and the alcohol is usually in the last aisle you come to, when you're tired and you'll buy anything just so that you can go home. But there's nothing to stop you starting at the far end and working back to the fruit and veg, is there? You can buy more bananas and tomatoes if you balance them on top of the rice and cans of beans, and they will still be edible when you get them home.

Make sure you identify your priority when you go shopping – is it health or entertainment?

Affirmations

Make up an Affirmation.

It should be a phrase that instantly conjures up a compelling picture of yourself, looking and feeling the way you want to be.

For example:

'I'm slim and getting slimmer.'

'I'm fit and getting fitter.'

'I'm becoming more of the person I want to be every day.'

If you don't fancy one of those, make up your own:

....

When you repeat your Affirmation, bring an image to mind of yourself being this way.

Make the image big, bright, bold and colourful; feel what it's like to have what you want.

Make a 'Me' movie with yourself as the star.

Practise this over and over, repeating your Affirmation as many times as possible each day.

Take the picture or movie you have made and take it with you wherever you go.

*ALL **Affirmations** sound silly at first. Start quietly and build them up. Don't worry at the beginning about whether you believe them.*

Think Positive, Speak Positive

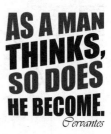

Be sure your thoughts become you. First your mind and then your body needs to learn and then practise for the goal you are moving towards.

Weight-loss starts in your mind. You now know how to be slimmer, fitter and healthier. You eat a healthy balanced diet and exercise regularly. And you think thin.

Many successful people owe their achievements to messages they constantly repeated to themselves over and over again. *'I will be famous, I will be rich...'* Steven Spielberg for one, Sylvester Stallone for another.

Many unsuccessful people also owe their failures to the compelling messages they've been running in their mind: *'I'm fat'*, *'I'm useless'*, *'I'm just not lucky'*, *'My face doesn't fit'*.

You get what you focus on and thoughts expand to fit the available space. So, as Emerson and Gandhi both said, it's a good idea to think about what you want, not what you don't want.

We take the miracle of thought for granted. There are limitations to what you can do with your body, but your mind has no limits at all. Whatever you can dream is waiting for you, so, continue to spend your time constructively, thinking about being the way you want to be.

An ideal time to repeat your **Affirmations** is when you're taking your **Fat-Burning Pills**. You've got a head start because you're using your body anyway. The more often you repeat your Affirmation to yourself, the easier it will be to believe and the more quickly you will reach your goals.

Repetition is the mother of all skill. If you tell yourself what you want over and over again, and vividly imagine it, you will move closer and closer to your **Outcome**.

...I look wonderful this morning...!

Bleep...

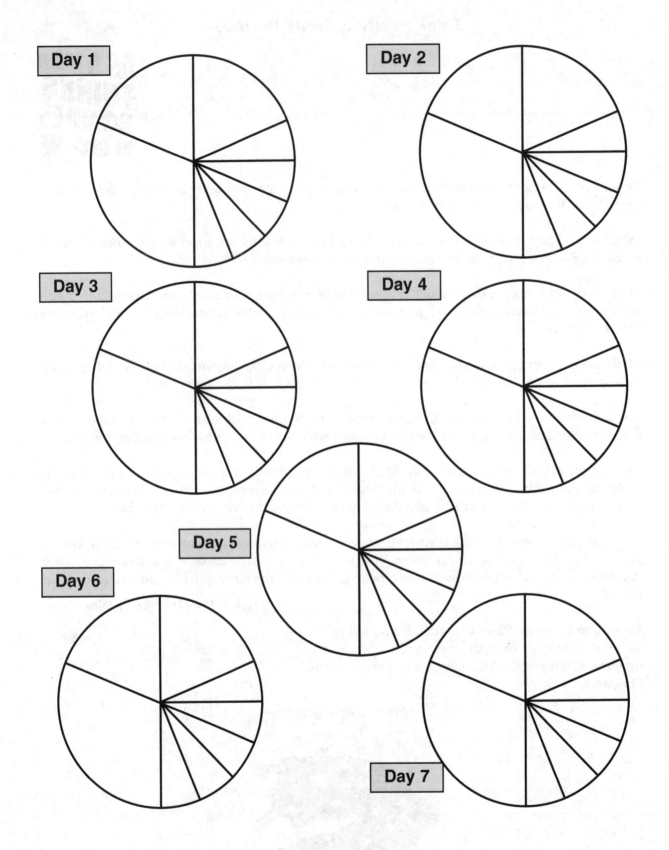

Next Week's Diary

You'll notice that I haven't given you an example of a **Food Diary** format this week because I think you will have got the hang of it by now. You've probably designed it to suit yourself and you can add as many different headings and categories as you like. Remember to include the **Hunger Scale**.

- Continue to note your feelings and log your exercise as well as the food you eat.

- Fill in the **Food Cake** and eat more of the foods you've been missing out on.

- Record how much good quality carbohydrate and fruit and vegetables you are eating.

- Write down how much more water you're drinking.

- Make a note of the exercise sessions when you use the Borg Scale and write down how many **Fat-Burning Pills** you are taking every day.

- Separate eating from your other activities whenever you can. Slow it down and savour it.

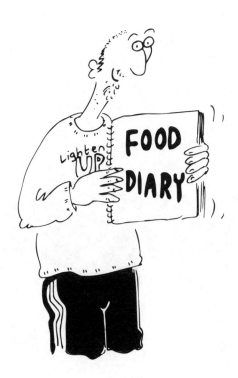

Slow Down!

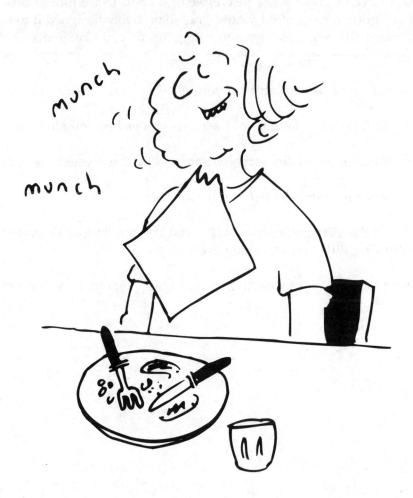

Put your knife and fork down between bites.

➡ Leave food on your plate occasionally. Maybe you do already, but if it's something you *never* do, it's very important. For some of us it's an ingrained habit, reinforced by some pretty important commands we were given long before we could understand them logically. Nobody could possibly ever get the right amount on their plate every time. If you never leave anything, there must be times when you're eating more than you're hungry for.

➡ Take time over your meals. Researchers at the University of Pennsylvania Medical School discovered that people who extend mealtimes by an average of four minutes, chewing more slowly and enjoying their food, burned up more body fat than the high speed eaters. Your brain needs about twenty minutes to get the signal that you've eaten enough.

Challenges

➡ Put your knife and fork down between bites and wait thirty seconds between mouthfuls. DON'T time it!

➡ *Think Before You Eat*.

➡ Use the **Changing Association With Food** strategy.

➡ **Think Before You Shop.**

➡ Set your **Outcomes.**

➡ Give yourself credit. Every time you do something that contributes to your success, pat yourself on the back. Do it.

➡ Use your **Affirmations**.

➡ Use the **Open Door** exercise.

➡ Respond to mistakes by learning and moving on.

➡ Cook some meals from the recipes at the end – or buy yourself a new cookbook.

➡ As usual, check through the chapter again to make sure you have done all the exercises.

Week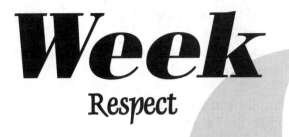
Respect

A couple of years ago, I was watching a friend play an important tennis match. Every time he hit a bad shot he swore at himself and, as the game continued, the abuse got louder. When he lost the second set he smashed his racket on the court. But his performance didn't improve; the madder he got, the more shots he missed.

After the game I went up to him and said: 'Ben, who were you calling an idiot just now?'

He gave me the traditional withering look. 'Me, of course; I'm not blaming anybody else. Don't tell me you couldn't see what complete rubbish I was.'

'What does talking to yourself like that do for you?' I asked him.

'I'm trying to get myself to play better, obviously,' he said, looking at me like I was an idiot.

'Didn't seem to be working, did it?'

Now, Ben's a teacher, and later, in the pub, I asked him: 'Is that how you motivate the kids, then, when they aren't doing well?'

'That's different,' he said. 'Kids have to be encouraged. What I generally do is get them to focus on what's working and do it more often. If I point out their bad shots, they seem to play them all the time.'

'Alright, then,' I said. 'Forget the kids. What if I come to you for help with my bowling? Are you going to yell abuse at me? I need to know!'

I eventually got him round to the idea that having one rule for the way he treated other people and a completely different one for himself was crazy. I even got him to give himself some encouragement. He had to pat himself on the back when he played well. And when he didn't, I got him to shake it off by either laughing at it or learning from it and being curious about what was happening.

When I saw him a few weeks later and asked for a progress report, he admitted that the new system took some getting used to. After all, patting yourself on the back in public takes courage. But then he went on to tell me that he was playing the best tennis he had ever played and that he felt relaxed and incredibly alert when he was on the court. He was beating players he had thought were out of his league. Most importantly though, *he was having fun.*

Last Week's Food Diary And Challenges

❖ Are you honouring your feelings? When you have negative emotions like sadness, guilt, anxiety and loneliness, don't bury them in food.

❖ Is the Borg scale helpful? And are you keeping up your minimum of fifteen minutes walking a day and filling up the **Fat Jar**?

❖ Have you been giving yourself credit for all the victories, large or small, over any old eating patterns you weren't really enjoying or which weren't useful any more?

❖ Is the **Hunger Scale** becoming automatic now?

❖ Are you using **Affirmations** and daydreaming, regularly and positively?

❖ Was it easy to leave food on your plate?

❖ How did you get on with putting your knife and fork down between mouthfuls?

❖ *Think Before You Eat* and **Think Before You Shop** soon become hard-wired, like the **Hunger Scale**.

❖ Did you Change Your Association with a particular food that's been dominating you?

❖ How many good quality carbohydrates, fruit and vegetables did you add to the **Food Cake**? Are you drinking more water?

❖ Are you setting **Outcomes** every day? And how you are responding to setbacks now as changes start to happen?

❖ Do you enjoy lingering over your meals a little more?

How Are You Doing?

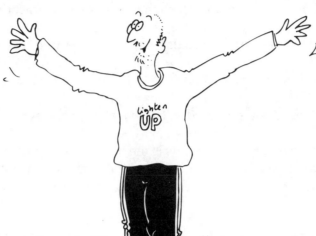

Now that you are into your sixth week, I'll be focusing more on food. But, food will never be the most important thing about losing weight. In fact, the reason why you haven't lost weight in the past may be because you've focused too much on it.

What matters, much more than what you eat, is how you treat yourself. In a word: respect. If you respect your body and your own good intentions, you are much more likely to succeed, whether it's in losing weight or winning a game of tennis. When you respect yourself, you are more likely to eat what your body needs and exercise regularly and you are more likely to have a positive self-image to work towards. You are definitely more likely to learn from your own mistakes and move on to success when you are prepared to give yourself a fair hearing.

So, forget about calling yourself names and start giving yourself more credit. It's one secret ritual you can be proud of and you can substitute it for the nightly weigh-in, now that you've got rid of your scales.

And, as you make changes, week by week, you will start to notice the domino effect. As you increase the activity in your daily routine, you may also see changes in both your lifestyle and your energy levels. Don't be afraid to congratulate yourself when these positive things start happening.

Now that you are getting into the routine of the **Food Diary**, you may be interested in the feelings associated with, when and what you eat, and how much better you start to feel about eating as you enjoy your food more.

I know some changes take a little longer than others. Sometimes it's the really simple things that seem to be the hardest. Leaving food on your plate, for example, is almost impossible for some people (although easy for others). Some of us hear some old messages replayed when we try to put a few potatoes in the bin, or give the fatty bits of meat to the dog.

In order to change, we have to challenge those beliefs we still live by, but which don't work for us any more. We are in a stronger position to stand up to our past if we are feeling strong and positive about ourselves and convinced of our own ability to succeed.

SAS Tactics

You can cope in difficult situations. Plan ahead and be prepared. Put together your own SAS (Sabotage Avoidance Strategies) plan. Here are a few that have been tried and tested by some friends of mine:

- Predict the danger points in a social situation. If you're not very assertive, don't be caught unawares. Rehearse some answers for when you get into an eating-pressure situation.

- Eat only special foods – go for the salad or sandwiches and leave the desserts.

- Eat slowly. Start last and make it last.

- Eat something before you go out; don't arrive at a special event starving.

- When you're at a party, remember, this is the only place and time when you can talk to this particular group of people – but you can eat peanuts at home anytime. Somebody in this room might change your life, with an idea, a job opportunity, a personal revelation or a new love affair.

- Sit down to eat. Then you'll be more aware of starting and finishing.

- Talk to other people about the food, praise the taste and style and presentation.

- Dance a lot. If nobody else is dancing, get them started.

- Offer to help in order to stay occupied.

- Take what you want from the buffet table and eat it somewhere else.

- If you're drinking alcohol, don't let anyone top up your glass. Wait until you've finished one before starting another. That way, you'll know how much of a hangover you're entitled to.

- When you've had enough, just stop and explain you're full.

- Remember, this is your life, your body and you decide what goes in it.

Think how good you will feel when you leave, knowing that you haven't overeaten.

When People Try To Make You Eat

Sometimes people will try to make you eat. They may have lots of different reasons for doing this and you can have fun tailoring your avoidance strategy to their motivation. Just ask yourself what these people really mean when they hold out that plate of mini spring rolls and say, 'Oh, go on, you have to try these, they're yummy'.

'I'm out to sabotage you.'
People with weight problems absolutely hate it when they see someone else being strong-minded. You are responsible for your own health and happiness, but not for their state of mind. So say, '*No*' and leave them to it.

'It's the only way I know to show I love you.'
Some people can only show affection freely through offering food. This is particularly true of older relatives and it requires a tactful response. After all, they may have lived through the war and know what it was like to eat bread and marrow jam for breakfast with no butter. If you see them often, tell them that you have a complicated food allergy and that you are likely to puff up and explode without warning if you eat anything the doctor hasn't prescribed. If you only see them every other Christmas explain that you got food poisoning yesterday and ask for a doggy bag to take home for when you're feeling better.

'It's the only way I know to ask you if you love me.'
Never mind the food; try just giving them a direct answer to the question. Like a hug.

'It's the only way I know to be sociable.'
Very often food covers a social problem. Some people aren't very good at conversation and they find it's less embarrassing to feed you than to try to talk to you. If you're confronted with someone like this, distract them by talking to *them*, preferably about something other than eating. Always be sure to praise what they've prepared, even if you're not eating much of it. You can comment on how it looks, and how long it must have taken – there's always something you can say without actually having to stuff yourself silly with it.

'I'm miserable, I'm going to overeat and I want company.'
This is a dangerous one. You feel sorry for the person and you know how they feel. Try getting them to talk instead of eat. If nothing will turn them from their self-destructive purpose, leave them to it. You may lose a friend. Temporarily. Eating with them won't help.

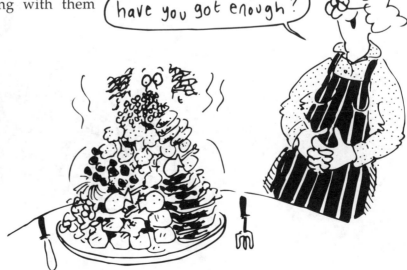

Calorie-saving Devices

What effect do labour-saving devices have on your life?

Did you know that the average British adult watches twenty-four hours of TV every week compared to thirteen hours in 1960?

Little Things Mean A Lot

Some sad person has worked out that you can burn an extra 132.3 calories a week by walking over to the TV five times a day instead of using your remote control. An even sadder person then calculated that this was true only for people whose TVs were twenty feet from their sofas. As this applies to such a small percentage of the population, I don't think that is useful information. In fact, I'll go further and say that calorie counting in general, whether it's calories in or calories out, is pretty futile.

You can't put the clock back and, if you've got a remote control, a washing machine and a dishwasher you might as well use them. In spite of the fact that twenty minutes of washing up apparently burns around 40 calories. Sorry, I promised not to do that.

Increasing your level of activity is what's important and there are far more interesting ways of getting movement into your life than washing up and scrubbing floors. So, do the things you've got to do (including washing up), with vim and vigour and then go out and do something for fun. The one area where you might consider abandoning convenience in the interests of exercise is travelling. A lot of us use cars and buses in situations when we could walk or ride a bike. It often doesn't make much difference time-wise, but, over time it will lose you pounds (and save you pounds as well).

Warning: *Labour-saving devices are also calorie-saving devices.*

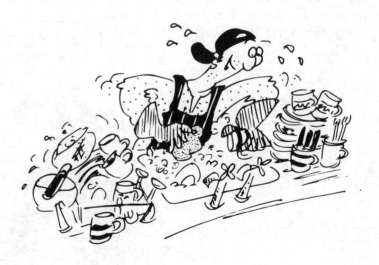

Saving Time For A Shorter Life

Having an idea of how active you are might make you aware that you spend large amounts of time not *doing* very much physically. Sitting in front of the TV, using the remote control, driving to work, putting the clothes in the washing machine and the dirty dishes in the dishwasher, buying ready meals and sitting in front of the VDU at work all day. So, OK, you may be mentally exhausted, but your body is *bored*.

What right do we have to neglect our bodies like that? No wonder they let us down.

According to Dr Nick Wareham at the Department of Community Medicine, the rise in obesity over the last twenty years can't be explained by calorie intake, which has been falling steadily. The real reason is that we have become far too sedentary – African villagers are three times as active as we are. A study of twelve thousand Finns in the European Journal of Clinical Nutrition found that they gained more weight through inactivity than through overeating.

It has become the norm to consume more energy than we use. If we really want to be slimmer we are going to have to increase our level of activity in everyday life. A study by the Health Education Authority indicated that two thirds of women aren't active enough to be healthy. And it's not just hearts and lungs that are being neglected, it's bones as well. Our grandparents might not have done the gym three times a week, but most of the population earned a living by physical hard work. What's more, washing, cooking and cleaning were done the hard way, and even social lives required effort in the days before cars, off-licences and videos.

The manufacturing industry is constantly encouraging us to buy more devices and ready-made products. We are being programmed to think it's a good idea to have lots of labour-saving, time-saving devices, which is fine if we're going to do something exciting with all the time we've saved. It's not fine if it leads us to spend even more of every twenty-four hours sitting down, because that's bad for your body and, if your body isn't happy, your mind won't be content.

We are constantly trying to save time, **but what are we saving it for?**

Do yourself a favour: get off your backside, be more active and start feeling great.

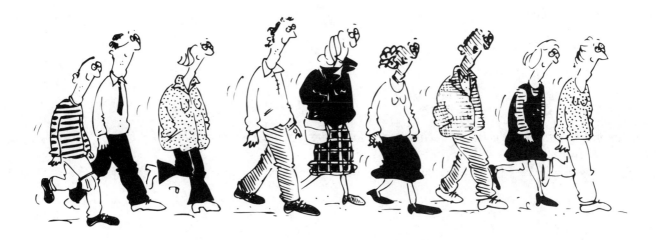

Exercise

And now, just so that you don't forget that food is only one part of the picture, I want you to think about something else: EXERCISE.

Give yourself five minutes and find a quiet place. Ask yourself these questions:

- What do you want to achieve?

- Is it your goal to be slimmer, fitter, happier, to feel better about yourself?

- If it is, what part does exercise play in achieving it?

- What do you want exercise to do for you?

- What are the benefits you get from exercising? How does it make you feel?

- What would it cost you if you didn't do any?

- How can you make your exercise even more enjoyable?
  - *Do it with a friend*
  - *Join a gym*
  - *Work with a trainer*
  - *Find a new way of exercising*
  - *Buy a piece of exercise equipment for your home*
  - *Take up a sport*
  - *Use an exercise video*

....

....

- How can you include even more activity in your daily life?
  - *Walk to work*
  - *Cycle to work*
  - *Walk at lunchtime*

I commit to being more active by including the following activity in my daily life:

....

....

Signed ....

Exercise

How well are you getting on with your exercise regime? How full is your **Fat Jar**?

When you enjoy exercise, you'll want to do it. We all find time to do the things we want to. *'I'm too busy'* is the most common reason people give for not exercising. But they won't be too busy to watch TV or go to the pub. The only way you will ever make exercise part of your life is when you enjoy it. And the only way you will ever be the size you want to be is by making exercise part of your daily routine.

Movement, activity, exercise, call it what you want, is the only way to become successfully slimmer forever. Exercise educates your body to burn fat.

Everyday
The secret is to sneak activity into everyday situations wherever you see the slightest opportunity: run up the stairs, walk up the escalator, walk to work, get a basket on your bike and cycle to the shops, throw away the remote control and walk over to the TV, choose a local that's not quite so local and, if you're thinking of buying a pet, make it a greyhound, not a goldfish.

A Little More
If all else fails, just take up walking briskly on a regular basis. Hardly imaginative, but highly effective. Plus you get to spend what you save on petrol as well as what's in the **Fat Jar**.

Exercise
Effective fat-burning activity is comfortable and continuous. Your breathing should be steady and audible, not laboured. Use the Borg scale to check you are exercising at level six to eight.

HELP!
If you want some help with motivation, why not exercise with a friend? – especially if you don't like exercising alone.

Or you could join a health club or get a personal trainer. Get professional advice and learn more about exercise so that you can constantly improve. This is especially important if you're an impatient personality and you want results instantly. Many people give up if they don't immediately get what they want when they want it.

Keep your bigger picture handy, to see the benefit of your exercise routine. If your goal is to become fitter, slimmer, and healthier and have loads of energy and vitality, what sort of role will exercise have in your vision of the future? Focus on activity giving you energy, making you feel good and releasing any tension or stress.

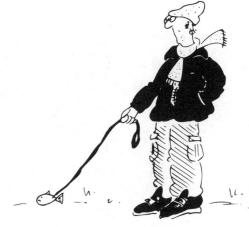

Treat Your Body With Respect

How do you behave when you're with someone you truly respect – a parent, teacher, mentor, priest, guru, leader, boss, colleague or friend? Would you give space, time, affection, even reverence? Surely you wouldn't irritate or upset the person you admire so much? That would be truly disrespectful.

Time to get the Diary out again – writing down your answers often clarifies them:

- Is your body worth respecting?

- If no, why not?

- If yes, why?

- Would you like to respect your body?

Tips for Treating Your Body With Respect

- If your body tells you you're thirsty, drink. If it tells you you're hungry, eat.

- Look after your body; spare part surgery has a long way to go.

- Say something nice to yourself when you wake up in the morning and when you sign off at night.

- Eat healthy, fresh food.

- Keep moving. That's what you were designed for. You know what happens to a bicycle chain when you don't look after your bike and use it regularly.

- There's more to rest than sleeping. Take some time out every day to breathe deeply and relax all your muscles.

- Cut down on stuff you don't enjoy, increase stuff you do and make the stuff you've got to do more fun.

Listen To Your Body

By this stage many of you have all the tools you need to live a healthy life. Even better, they are becoming second nature now and you can pick them up whenever you need them.

So your focus will shift now. Away from understanding the tools and healthy eating plans towards listening to your body. Giving it the right things at the right time. Living in balance and equilibrium with yourself.

Your body knows genetically, from birth, how to keep you at the perfect weight. It may not be *your* idea of the perfect weight because icons of beauty are rarely average in height, weight or appearance. So most of the population can *never* naturally look like the people they most admire. *The Body Shop* is beginning to recognise this and uses some images which look more like real people. Trust your body. The perfect weight that you can be may not be catwalk thin, but it won't be Robbie Coltrane either.

Babies won't eat when they're not hungry but, over the years, you've learned to eat for reasons other than hunger. Your body never stopped sending you messages about how to eat, but you stopped listening.

If you're a leopard, you can't suddenly decide to make a fashion statement by joining up your spots and making them into stripes. You can't fight your genetic design. But although you *know* that, most people don't want to accept it. Normal eating and dieting are incompatible. Normal eaters eat regular meals. They don't worry about food and their diet tends to be very varied. They don't worry about their body weight either.

Life is for living and every day is full of potential that needs to be realised. You have more potential than ever before and those new daily habits you've been playing around with will give you the feedback you need to stay happy and balanced.

So, loosen up a little, be flexible with your day. Listen to what your body is telling you and act accordingly.

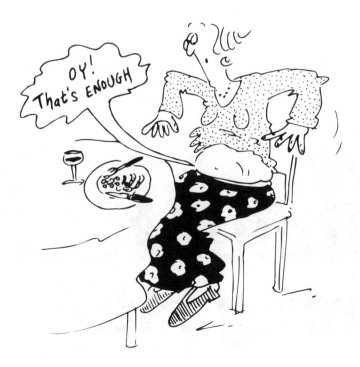

How Much Fat?

Recommended Daily Intake: 2 servings for large, medium and small persons

One Food Cake serving is:

> 1 tablespoon of oil, margarine, butter
> 4 tablespoons of cream
> Handful of nuts
> Small handful of seeds
> 4 teaspoons of peanut butter
> Small bag of crisps
> Small portion of chips
> Couple of biscuits

- Use skimmed or low fat milk, non-fat or low fat yoghurt.

- Cut down on or cut out cakes, chocolates, sweets and crisps.

- Eat meat in modest portions, choose lean cuts and limit the use of processed meat.

- Use olive oil when you're cooking, instead of saturated fat.

- Eat plenty of vegetables; they are a good supply of fibre, vitamins and minerals as well as being low in fat and having no cholesterol.

- Trim off the fat before cooking meat and remove skin.

- Use non-stick pans and olive oil for frying.

- Substitute low fat or non-fat plain yoghurt for sour cream or mayonnaise.

- Grill or bake meat instead of frying.

- Eat plenty of fresh fruit.

- Eat more fish – it's low in saturated fat, cholesterol and calories and it's a good source of protein, B vitamins and zinc.

The more **active** you are, the more **efficient** you will become at **burning fat.**

How Much Energy?

How much fat should you eat?

It depends on your lifestyle.

The human body has a really easy time converting fat into fat which is a valuable source of energy and protects against heat loss. It contains twice the calories (nine per gram) of either protein or carbohydrate. So, if you plan to walk across the Antarctic, towing your own sledge, it should definitely be the main part of your diet.

Sedentary, non-Eskimos tend to see fat as an enemy, which is realistic. Especially since about 60% of fats are hidden in foods like cakes, chocolates, biscuits and crisps and we don't always realise how much we're eating. Once we cut down on, or cut out these foods, our fat intake is lowered quite substantially.

But don't try to cut it out altogether. That's quite dangerous because fat contains vitamins A, D, E and K that are essential for a healthy body. It also protects our vital organs; it's a valuable source of energy and provides flavouring for many foods. And we need fat to burn fat.

It really comes down to the amount and type of fat we eat.

There are three types of fat:

- **Saturated fat**, which is solid at room temperature and comes primarily from meat and dairy products. High consumption of this is associated with heart disease and it is recommended that we eat only very small quantities.

- **Monounsaturated fats** are found in olive and peanut oils.

- **Polyunsaturated fats,** which are generally liquid or soft at room temperature, are found mainly in sunflower, corn, soya bean oils and in some fish oils.

All these fats contain the same amount of calories, but polyunsaturated and monounsaturated fats are better for us.

Follow the guidelines on the left to check your fat intake.

Eating Protein

Fish, Meat, Poultry and Soya/Tofu

Recommended Daily Intake: 2 servings for large, medium and small persons

One Food Cake Serving is: 3oz lean meat, poultry, fish, soya or tofu

- Choose lean meat, fish, and poultry without skin, and prepare meat in low fat ways by trimming it and not frying it.

- Increase the proportion of fish and chicken rather than red meat and dairy food in your protein allowance.

Beans and Lentils

Recommended Daily Intake: 2 servings for large, medium and small persons

One Food Cake Serving is: 1 cup of cooked beans or lentils

There are many different types of lentils and beans. It's better to buy fresh ones wherever possible, but dried ones are good too. You can add them to soups, casseroles or just about any meal including salads. Some people prefer them to meat, and lots of people find them an acceptable substitute in some of their meals.

Chick peas
Kidney beans (must be very well cooked)
Lentils
Black eye beans
Lima beans
Butter beans
French beans

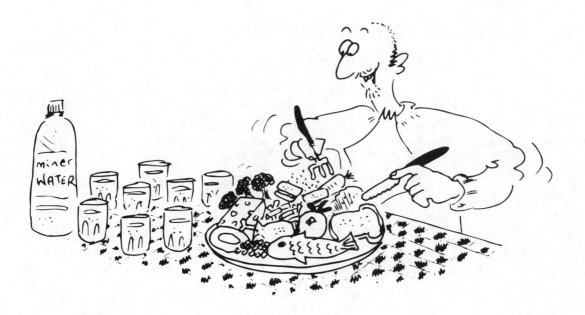

Protein

Fish, Meat, Poultry, Soya/Tofu, Beans and Lentils

Every cell in the body has to have protein. It's needed for the growth and repair of everything from muscles and bones to hair and fingernails. The best way of getting enough of it is to make sure you have a variety of sources in your diet, but eating too much of it is counter-productive because the body can't store it for later.

Herbivore or Carnivore?

Fish, meat and poultry contain all the high quality proteins the body needs to maintain good health, although many experts believe that meat is not essential and that we can live quite easily without it. On the other hand, vegetable proteins, including soya, usually lack some parts of the essential proteins, so vegetarians need to pay close attention to their diets to make sure they are getting balanced nutrition.

Vegetable Sources of Protein

Since some meat has a high fat content and eating a lot of red meat is often linked to heart disease, it's a good idea to include some vegetarian sources of protein in your diet. Fortunately, there are plenty of good quality protein sources in cereals (wheat, oats, rice and bread), in eggs and dairy products and in pulses (peas, beans and lentils), nuts, seeds and potatoes.

Beans, including soya, tofu and lentils are particularly good. If you eat them with a grain such as rice or bread – beans on toast or lentil dhal with rice – you'll be getting all the proteins you need. They also contain both soluble and insoluble fibre which is great for your health in other ways.

Apart from the sweetened baked beans in the full English breakfast, many people never eat pulses at all. People who do eat them regularly generally love them and cook very creatively with them. But, if you're one of the majority and don't think they are real food, give them a try. Buy some chick peas, broad beans, black-eyed beans, mung beans, green and red lentils, red kidney beans or borlotti beans and experiment with some of the recipes at the end of the book.

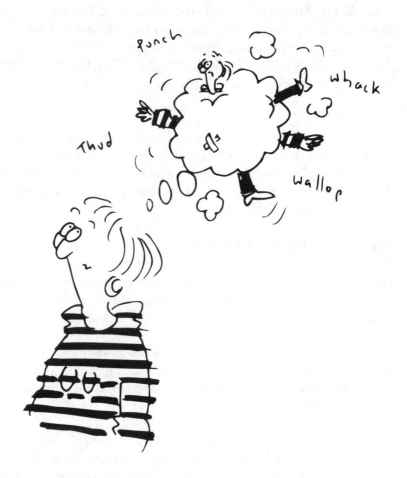

If you can't be good to yourself, your chances of success are slimmer than you'll ever be.
~ Hedera Foley, *silent screen star*

Health Food For The Mind

We all know that *we are what we eat*. A fresh, healthy, balanced diet is a necessary provision for the journey to becoming slimmer and living a long life full of vitality and energy. We've spent too long putting food into our bodies when we aren't physically hungry. To make matters worse, the food we're putting in is often full of sugar, fat, chemicals, preservatives and additives; it can poison and confuse our bodies. Many dieters are so worried about calories and fat that they forget to look for all the other nasties. Before we take the first steps towards our slimmer, fitter selves, we need to start treating ourselves with more respect.

Now, if we are prepared to be kinder to our bodies, shouldn't we also think twice about the poison we constantly feed our minds? Health food for thought? Yes, it's about taking control over our mental states.

A good way to get better acquainted with your inner world is by listening to your internal dialogue. This may feel strange at first because you are bringing into awareness an automatic process.

Giving yourself a hard time is like systematically ingesting small doses of arsenic; in the end, it's a killer. There's no point in filling your mind with junk: *'I'm stupid'*, *'I can't do this'*, *'I'm fat'*, *'He won't like me'*...

BE NICE TO YOURSELF

Our culture has taught us to be our own toughest critics. We are obsessed with problems. The most popular television programmes are soap operas, current affairs, news and disaster programmes. When people get together they talk about what's wrong with their lives. Their house is too small, their salary is too low, their street is too noisy, their car is too old. It's more acceptable to talk about your problems than your triumphs. That's called boasting. Next time you walk down a busy street, take a look at how many people have smiling faces and how many more look blank or miserable.

The most important thing to remember is that *you get what you focus on*. Focus on feeling good for no reason at all. Look for positive things in your life and you'll get more of them.

Getting To Know Yourself Better

Nobody can be exactly like me.
Sometimes
even I have trouble doing it.
— Tallulah Bankhead, actress

For the next couple of weeks, pay attention to your internal dialogue, listen to it, be curious about how you talk to yourself.

- What do you say to yourself?

- How do you treat yourself?

- What messages do you give yourself?

- What do you talk to your friends about?

- What do you read?

- What do you watch?

Where is your attention – are you fascinated by problems, or by how to solve them?

- If you start to give yourself a hard time, stop it.

- If you hear that voice telling you you're stupid, turn around and tell it to shut up.

- When you talk to yourself, be polite, be gentle, be nice.

- Give yourself encouragement.

- Be kind to yourself.

- Be your own best friend.

If you make a mistake, learn from it, laugh at it, leave it behind.

Being Your Own Best Friend

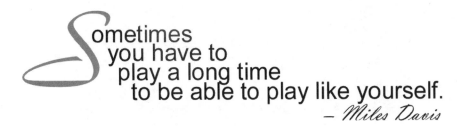

Sometimes
you have to
play a long time
to be able to play like yourself.
– Miles Davis

We say the first sign of madness is talking to yourself. If that's true we're all mad because we all do it. But, because we don't usually do it out loud, nobody notices, not even us.

If I asked you what your favourite colour is or what you had for dinner last night, you would immediately be answering the questions in your mind. I want you to become more aware of your internal dialogue.

Remember Ben and the game of tennis? In my life as a sports trainer, I've seen a lot of people screaming verbal abuse at themselves (and sometimes at me) *and it only ever makes the situation worse.*

I have worked with so many people who want to be slimmer, and a lot of them discourage themselves in just the same way. They all want to look good and feel good but they sabotage themselves with bad eating habits and giving themselves a hard time.

'I shouldn't have eaten that … I'm so stupid … I should have taken more exercise …I can't do it … I've got no will power…'

That's what I call beating yourself up mentally. As often as not, this is the kind of social response that we've learned from parents and teachers. The people I know who have successfully become slimmer have stopped battling with themselves. They've learned to be kind and accept themselves for who they are. They changed and so can you.

Pay attention to your dialogue and start to free yourself from criticising and giving yourself a hard time.

Use the exercise on the left to get you started with your new friendship.

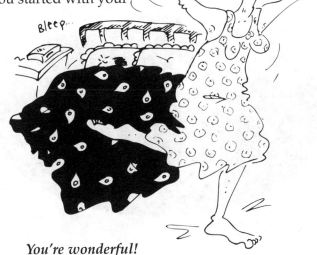

You're wonderful!

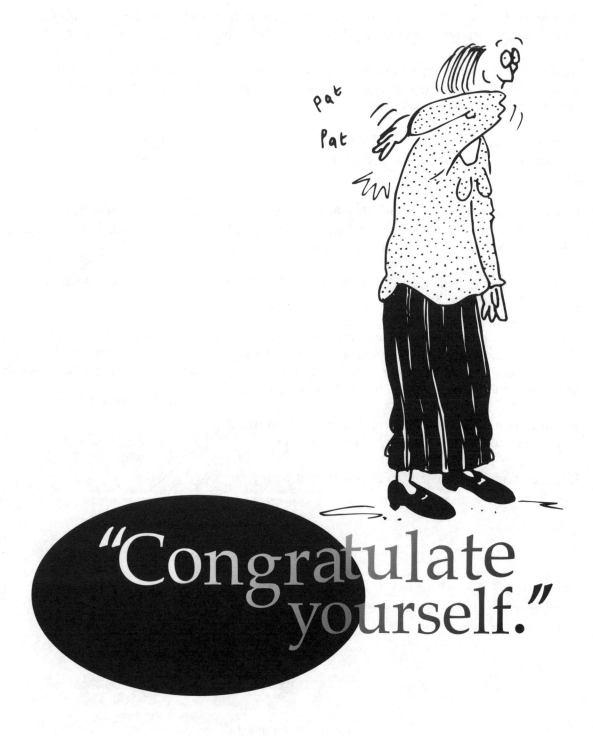

Next Week's Diary

- Note where you are on the **Hunger Scale** before every meal.

- *Think Before You Eat* and, every so often, write down the food you reject as well as the food you select.

- Leave something on your plate sometimes, when you realise you're full. And when you do, record it in the diary.

- Use your **Food Cake** to get some feedback about whether you are eating a balanced diet.

- Continue to record how much water you drink.

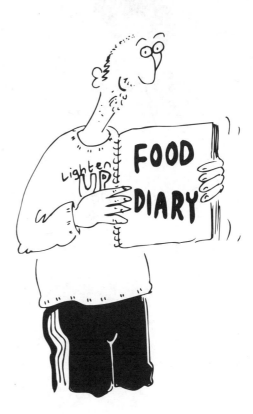

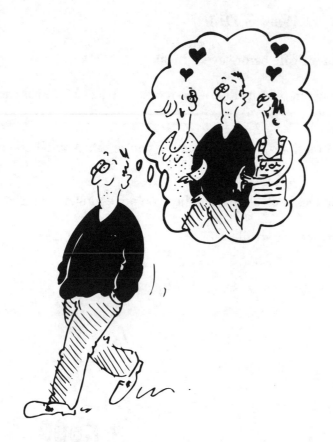

Go confidently in the direction of your dreams!
Live the life you've imagined.

Henry David Thoreau.

➠ Continue to take your **Fat-Burning Pills**.

➠ Look at new ways of increasing your activity levels.

➠ Look at the back of the book and treat yourself to some new recipes.

➠ Try out some Displacement Activities to block your eating response.

➠ Be your own best friend.

➠ Listen to your body and treat yourself with respect.

➠ Live your **Outcomes**.

➠ Give yourself credit.

➠ Experiment with the **Hunger Scale** half-way through a meal as well as at the beginning.

➠ Respond to setbacks by treating them as learning opportunities.

➠ Look to eat good sources of fat and protein.

➠ Remember you need health food for your body as well as your mind.

➠ And, as usual, make sure you've done *ALL* the exercises on the left.

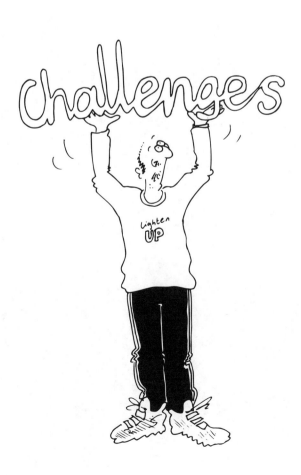

Week
Dancing Space

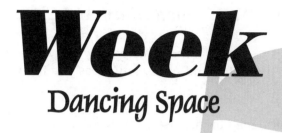

I met my friend Lewis the other week – I hadn't seen him for months and I hardly recognised him. 'You must have lost three stone,' I said as I took my drink over to his table. 'How did you do that? Tell me about it and I'll buy you another drink.'

But he was already getting up to leave. 'Sorry, Pete, I'll catch up with you later, I'm coaching the junior rugby and I'm running late.'

As the door slammed behind him, I looked at his glass – it was a half and he'd left some of it. He obviously had other priorities and it was showing on his waistline. I remembered the last time I'd seen him in the same pub. He'd been propping up the bar complaining that he wouldn't be able to go for a curry at closing time because he was on yet another diet. 'You spend more time thinking about food than you spend eating it,' I told him. 'Apart from the fact that it's really boring for everybody else, have you ever thought of all the things you could do if you just went out and got a life?'

I realised that must be exactly what he'd done.

How much of your life do you spend doing things you don't really want to do, just to save yourself from doing other things you want to do even less? Life's full of hard choices and, for committed negative thinkers, most of those choices are between things we know we aren't going to enjoy very much and things we think we aren't going to enjoy at all.

Why eat food you aren't really tasting, when you aren't really hungry? You must really want to avoid writing that report, cleaning the loo, or phoning the bank manager!

Or maybe you just know you want something, but you don't know what. And food's the easy answer – after all, everybody has to eat.

And then, when you've filled in enough time with eating, you can waste a whole lot more by going to diet classes and counting calories. In fact, gaining weight and trying to lose it can keep you so busy that you never will have time to re-write your CV, or visit your auntie or complete your tax return. When it comes to Displacement Activities, eating's a real winner.

Do you really want to sort this out? What are you going to do with all that time you've freed up? You don't have to spend it all on voluntary work or cleaning out the fridge; you could have some fun with it as well. Look up old friends, give a party, take up a new sport, or go out dancing.

As one lady said at a Lighten Up workshop recently: 'I haven't found my dancing space yet – but I know what I'm looking for.'

Last Week's Food Diary And Challenges

There were a lot of things to bear in mind when you were writing your **Food Diary** last week. Here's the checklist. Run through it and notice any areas you found particularly interesting and any you didn't record.

- ❖ The **Food Cake** is designed to increase your awareness of your eating patterns.

- ❖ Are you recording your feelings about eating and before eating?

- ❖ The **Hunger Scale**.

- ❖ Thinking Before You Eat.

- ❖ Leaving some food on your plate.

- ❖ Recording how much water you drink.

- ❖ Taking **Fat-Burning Pills**.

- ❖ Looking at new ways of increasing your activity levels.

- ❖ Being your own best friend.

- ❖ Listening to your body and treating yourself with respect.

- ❖ Setting up and achieving your **Outcomes** every day.

- ❖ How are you coping with your mistakes now? Or are you starting to regard them as learning opportunities?

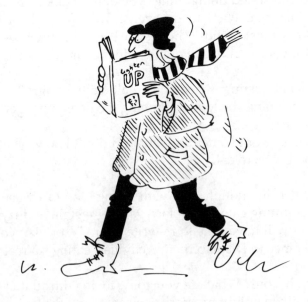

How Are You Doing?

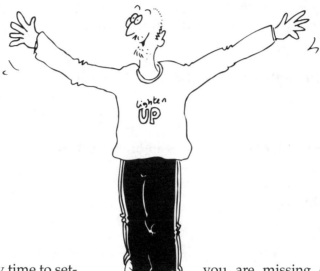

Give your mind and body time to settle into a new way of living. It's time to consider new ways of seeing things, new attitudes and new methods of self-management.

I asked you to be aware of a lot of things last week. Some of them will be ideas, or techniques, that you're taking for granted and doing automatically. There will be a few that you don't get along with and maybe aren't right for you yet. And there will be some that you're still working on.

Take the **Food Diary** and the **Food Cake** for example. They can be complementary and you might find it's useful to run both together, for a while at least. Or perhaps you prefer to record your eating patterns on the **Food Cake** and use the **Food Diary** more creatively. You could tailor it to the issues which seem most important to your own life and your own future.

The **Food Cake** is specially designed to show you whether you could have a more varied diet. Have you found any foods you are missing out on? This isn't about denial or deprivation, it's about meeting your body's needs for health, strength and fitness. If there are some foods you just can't put inside you, think around them a bit. What might you substitute that falls into the same category? Perhaps some new recipes would help – look at the back of the book.

It may be that you are learning some interesting things about how your feelings and your state of mind are relevant to your eating patterns. When you write things down and see them in black and white, you often notice things that you missed before. And, as you become more and more aware, you will also start to feel much more in control of your eating.

Finally, and very importantly, give yourself credit when you change a habit that has been limiting your life for years. And give yourself that pat on the back every time you recognise the difference between being hungry and thirsty, or just plain bored and fed up.

Sugarholics Alert!

Answer the following questions to find out whether you are a *sugarholic*.

I never have cravings for cakes, chocolates, sweets, soft drinks or biscuits.

T r u e/F a l s e

I can go for a day or so without eating any of the above.

T r u e/F a l s e

I can always stop after eating one sweet or biscuit or a single piece of chocolate.

T r u e/F a l s e

I can have a cupboard full of sweet snacks and not eat them.

T r u e/F a l s e

I rarely drink soft drinks.

T r u e/F a l s e

I never add sugar to tea, coffee, cereal or strawberries and raspberries.

T r u e/F a l s e

I don't automatically reach for something sweet to finish off a meal.

T r u e/F a l s e

There are times when I don't have any sweet treats in the house.

T r u e/F a l s e

If you answer *'False'* to three or more of these questions, you may well be sugar sensitive or addicted to the stuff.

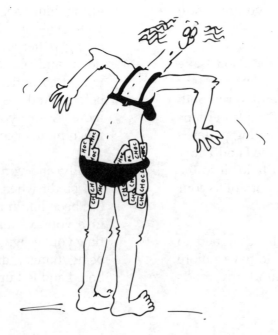

Sugar

What foods do you go for when you are lacking energy? What foods do you crave?

The question is, are you a sugarholic? Answer the questions on the left to help you find out.

Whether you are sugar sensitive or not, you might want to know that a number of recent studies have highlighted the dangers of excessive sugar consumption. Nasa Scientist, Dr William Grant is quoted as saying, 'People ... are not being told by the medical system that sugar is one of the big problems; they are unwilling to think of it as a killer.' The powerful sugar industry is widely blamed for the fact that many of the studies on the dangers of sugar consumption are not widely publicised.

Our bodies need two teaspoons of blood sugar at any one time in order to function properly. This can quite easily be taken through the digestion of complex sugars, brown rice, pasta, etc. as well as from protein and fat. Every bit of refined sugar you eat confuses your body and throws it out of balance. Yet sugar consumption in Britain has risen by 31% since 1980 and the average person eats 1.25 – 2lbs per week.

One of the biggest problems is the amount of 'hidden' sugar in pre-prepared and processed foods. Even so-called health foods, particularly those which boast a low fat content, often contain alarming amounts of sugar. A well-known breakfast bran cereal, for example, is 22% sugar and a famous diet drink is 61.9% sugar – higher than many brands of sweet biscuits and cakes.

Sweet and High

Sugars, whether brown or white, supply only empty calories with no nutritional value at all. It doesn't matter whether it's sucrose, fructose, glucose, lactose or maltose – it's a complete fallacy that one type of sugar is better for you than another. The only difference is that when they are eaten in their natural form such as fructose in fruit, they can supply many necessary vitamins and minerals as well as energy.

Sugar, like excessive fat, is a major disrupter of healthy eating. It's high in calories and it's also linked to diabetes, obesity, heart disease, migraines, low immunity, skin disorders, yeast overgrowth (candida) and, of course, tooth decay.

How Sweet Do You Need To Be?

Recommended Daily Intake: 2 servings for large, medium and small persons

One Food Cake serving is: 1 tablespoon of sugar, honey or jam

Sugar cravers may suffer from headaches, pains in the joints, fatigue and a bloated stomach. If you think it might be a problem for you, try cutting back on the amount you eat and see if you feel better.

Guidelines for Cutting Out Sugar

Gradually cut down on the amount of sugar added to food and drinks. Substitute with fruit.

Buy reduced or sugar-free versions of food and drinks – like sugar-free baked beans.

When baking, try and halve the sugar or use fruit or fresh juice for sweetening.

Beware of anything ending in 'ose' on food labels. Some foods may have up to four or five different types of sugar in them. But they are all the same thing – refined sugar.

Check all your food labels. You would be surprised at how much and how often sugar sneaks into food and it's all empty added calories.

White grapes and dried fruits are excellent for staving off sugar cravings. They are high in sugar, but also high in nutritional value.

Try to buy foods sweetened with juices or fruit.

Visit your local health shop. They have loads of healthy sweet treats. Beware though, as they also have loads of unhealthy sweet treats. Always check the labels, even in health stores.

When you have the urge for something sweet, ask yourself, *'Is this hunger or a craving?'* If it's a craving, do something else. Cravings come in waves, they build up and die down. Ride the wave.

Brush your teeth after sugary snacks.

Sugar And Fat

Sugar adds nothing to our diet. Fat, on the other hand, is essential – although a lot of people eat more of it than they need.

Cutting back on both of these could result in a much healthier diet; one that will help you to be slimmer, fitter and healthier, as well as reducing the risk of a lot of illnesses and longer-term physical malfunctions and discomforts.

Thirty years ago, obesity was less common. Many people ate more than we do now, but they also took more exercise. And the food they ate was more natural, with a higher proportion of fruit and vegetables and less pre-packed, chemically created products. The amount of fat and sugar in most people's diet was considerably lower than it is now.

What happens when we eat sugar and fat together?

When you eat a bar of chocolate or a triple layer fudge cake, there is a sudden explosion of pleasure on your taste buds, but it's short-lived. Your fat cells are immediately filled and your blood vessels are eventually left coated and clogged. A sugar hit puts a great strain on your regulatory system because sugar is absorbed so fast into the bloodstream.

It's like a selfish action which causes pain to a friend. You upset them, then you leave them with the bad feelings to sort out. When you eat sugar, your body is left to repair the damage you've caused by your craving for instant pleasure.

Fat and sugar mixes are highly refined and (as in shop-bought cakes) often loaded with chemicals.

This combination doesn't satisfy hunger so you don't know when you've had enough.

You can eat a lot of calories in this form without feeling full, which is why people often say they haven't eaten much – they don't think they have!

The fat and sugar combination activates huge amounts of digestive enzymes which make short work of your snack and send messages to the brain requesting more food. Most people can't eat just one chocolate, and after a fat and sugar snack you may feel even hungrier.

If you put the wrong octane petrol in your car, it won't run very well and you'll be causing long-term damage. If you try to run your body on cream buns and biscuits you're putting it under tremendous strain as you pound on the pounds. It's going to be less reliable and performance will suffer. And, if it breaks down completely, you can't replace it.

Convenience Foods

It's hot and there's lots of it…

Ask yourself, *'What am I going to do with the time I save on preparing this meal?'* Is it time worth saving? Or could you have just as much fun in the kitchen?

If you really need to save that time, ask how much longer it would take you to make yourself a healthy sandwich, or wash some salad, open a tin of tuna, or peel a banana. A proper meal doesn't necessarily have to be cooked. There's a saying about bad food in our family: *'At least it's hot and there's lots of it'*.

Make your own fast food – there are some really rapid-to-prepare recipes that taste a lot better than anything you can buy. I've included some of them at the end of this book.

If you are going to eat ready-made meals, why not add an extra portion of vegetables, or a salad. You might possibly even add an easy complex carbohydrate such as brown rice or a wholemeal bread roll.

When you eat at a junk food restaurant, skip the melted cheese and mayonnaise.

Some fast food places even have healthier alternatives now – including salad bars. Look out for them.

Always run *Think Before You Eat* and check out how that food is going to make you feel after you've eaten it.

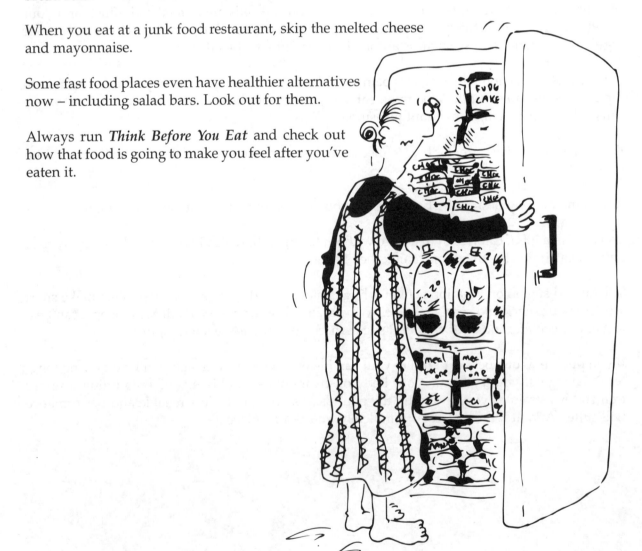

Faster Fat

Technological advances have increased the quality and range of convenience meals that are now available. We can get fat faster than ever before and with the most minimal expenditure of energy. We don't even have to collect our takeaways now that home delivery is available just about everywhere.

Vacuum packed or frozen, pre-cooked, microwaveable, meal-type foods are in all the shops. There's no excuse for bread and cheese and an apple for supper when you can pick up three courses from the corner shop on your way home from the station. In fact there are some things we just don't bother to prepare at home any more – when did you last make a hamburger? Assuming mad cows haven't put you off the idea altogether.

You can buy luxury convenience meals with really fancy packaging, or low-budget versions that you have to take care not to confuse with the cat treats. If you're working long hours, or you're trying to run a home, raise a family and study for your degree at the same time, they can be very appealing.

OK, so life's too short to stuff a mushroom, as Shirley Conran once said, but at least you knew what you were stuffing the mushroom with. As the study on sugar consumption that I mentioned earlier pointed out, there is a much higher proportion of sugar in almost every convenience food than we would ever put into a similar recipe we made at home. The reason for this is that it's much more cost effective to make something palatable by adding sugar (and salt) than by adding more of the expensive, fresh ingredients. Regardless of whether or not they are masquerading as complete meals, these easy meals are not usually an adequate source of vegetables or complex carbohydrates.

Fast food restaurants and takeaways are becoming more and more popular, especially with children. There is more variety and the food quality is better now than it was ten years ago. But they still don't measure up very well nutritionally. A typical cheeseburger and chips with apple pie and a large cola contains between 1100 and 1200 calories. And a lot of those calories come from saturated fats and sugar. The cola alone (besides colouring, chemicals and caffeine) contains around seven teaspoons of sugar. If your diet relies heavily on these foods you may not be getting enough vitamins, minerals and fibre.

Fast foods also crowd out fresh fruit and vegetables. Although the typical takeaway is high in saturated fat, salt and sugar and low in fibre, I still see more people snacking on fries than on fruit.

Getting What You Want

The questions you ask yourself have a major effect on the quality of your life.

- Do you have certain emotions on a daily basis that you don't like?

- Did you know that these emotions grow out of the questions you ask yourself?

- What happens when you say to yourself: *'Why am I so fat?'* Perhaps you get answers like *'Because you eat so much,'* or *'Because you have no self-control.'*

If you ask yourself negative questions your brain will come up with negative answers. If you constantly run this depressing stuff in your mind, you're going to make yourself feel bad.

Saying, *'Why does this always happen to me?'* won't empower you. It tips you into an endless loop of focusing on what isn't working in your life. It will depress you or whip you into a frenzy, but it isn't going to spur you into positive, affirmative action.

Just suppose, instead of asking questions like, *'Why can't I ever stick with a diet?'* you were to ask ones like:

'What's great about what I am doing?'
'How can I become slimmer right now?'
'What can I do that will start me on the road to becoming slimmer?'
'What do I need to do to make sure that I have a great day?'

Positive questions get positive answers. You could go a step further and ask:

'How can I become slimmer and enjoy the process?'
'How am I going to feel when I've been for a walk and I'm soaking in a hot bath?'
'What are the benefits I get from being slimmer, fitter and healthier?'
'How does eating a healthy balanced diet make me feel good?'

What a concept! Your brain will happily search for a quality answer because if you give it half a chance it will do anything to avoid pain and gain pleasure.

What you focus on is what you get. By asking yourself empowering questions, you begin to create possibilities.

Ask And You Shall Receive

Half the people who buy a computer use only a quarter of its capacity. Most people who buy sports cars don't drive them to within more than three-quarters of their potential performance (fortunately).

You're Amazing

We were all born with a computer more powerful than anything we could buy and we use much less than a quarter of it most of the time. We don't use our brains and we often neglect our bodies too. Every one of us is a more sophisticated and highly-tuned machine than the highest performance cars on the road – and we don't even bother to look after ourselves properly or use the best fuel.

The brain is like a sponge, always soaking in information. Unfortunately, most people take in too much negativity because their attention is focused on problems, on what's not working.

Think of one of your role models. It might be somebody richer or more successful, somebody with a bigger car or a lower golf handicap. Or it might just be somebody slimmer. What's the difference between you and your role model? Is it really just the luck of the genetic lottery, or, does it have more to do with your beliefs about yourself?

It doesn't matter whether it's hip size or happiness that's important to you. The winners in life are usually the people who have learned to use their mind and body on full power all the time and not skimp on the maintenance. Of course, we don't come with a User's Manual, we have to write our own. Which is what the **Food Diary** is all about.

You can waste brainpower by running low-grade software all the time. If the only screensaver you have is a line, which floats around saying *'I must lose some weight'*, this may be a sign that your software needs upgrading. Install a positive message and you might get a positive result.

If you must ask yourself leading questions, at least make sure they are leading you in the right direction. Asking yourself encouraging questions will help you to become even more resourceful and empowered. We all talk to ourselves all the time but we don't bother to edit what we say. We all need some encouragement – and the surest way to get it is to build it into our own brains.

Dairy Product, Nuts And Seeds

Recommended Daily Intake: 2 servings for large, medium and small persons

One Food Cake serving is: 1 egg
2oz low fat cheese
1 cup non-fat milk, ½ cup semi-skimmed milk
½ cup low fat yoghurt

- Use skimmed or semi-skimmed milk.

- Eat low fat cheese.

- Eat live yoghurt instead of ice cream, milk shakes and yoghurt with added sugar.

- Eat only one egg yolk in a serving.

- It is best to spread out your servings of dairy foods rather than eating them all in one sitting. And watch out for the hidden sugars as well as the fats.

- **Nuts and Seeds**

- Roasted ones tend to be acidic and heavily salted so it's best to eat them fresh.

- Most people know there are more than peanuts to choose from, but how many of us regularly snack on the full range?

Almonds
Brazils
Cashews
Coconut
Macadamias
Pecans
Pine nuts
Pistachios
Walnuts
Filberts
Hazelnuts

…as well as pumpkin, sesame, sunflower and poppy seeds. They are all very good for you, but don't pig out – they take a lot of digesting.

Dairy Product, Nuts And Seeds

Dairy Foods

These are a good source of protein and carbohydrate but they also contain lots of fat and they are high in cholesterol. Go for the ones that have a low fat content, otherwise you might use up all your daily fat servings in one go.

Dairy foods are a good source of vitamin A, vitamin D and calcium. Vitamins A and D are essential for the development and growth of skin, bones and teeth. Calcium is an essential mineral for good health. Roughly 2% of the body is calcium, most of which is teeth and bones.

If you are worried about eating too many dairy foods but you want to be sure you are getting enough calcium, remember that tofu made with the setting agent calcium chloride is the richest non-dairy source of calcium.

Seeds and Nuts

Nuts and seeds are high in calories, but not empty calories by any means. They are another underrated and neglected source of protein and vitamins. Their reputation as real nourishment suffered when they became commonly used as a cocktail snack, and a lot of people still won't eat them because they think they are too fattening.

Well, so they are, but they are also very high in nutritional value so, as long as you eat them when you are physically hungry, they are good for you as well as tasting great.

Seeds and nuts make great healthy snacks. And they are also very easy to add to meals. Pumpkin, sesame and sunflower seeds taste wonderful on a whole range of vegetable dishes and salads.

DON'T eat them if you have a nut allergy.

Healthy Cooking

- Eat plenty of vegetables.

- Grill rather than fry.

- Choose white meat and fish in preference to red meat.

- Reduce the amount of added sugar.

- Reduce the amount of added cream and high fat cheese.

- Trim the fat and the skin from meat.

- Reduce the amount of oil you use in cooking and dressings.

- Roast vegetables (you don't really need fat).

- Roast meat and let the fat drain.

- Reduce the amount of added salt.

- Steam vegetables.

- Separate the fat from the juice to make gravy.

- Check the recipes at the back of the book for ideas.

Healthy Cooking

If you always do what you've always done...

The secret of change is to do something differently from the way you were doing it before. Slimming is no exception. So, if you've counted calories before, cut out fat/carbohydrate/protein/puddings before or brought yourself to the edge of a heart attack by over-exercising:

you already know it doesn't work.

It's time to do something different. And the first step is to give yourself a shot of pleasure to get you going. View yourself in a positive light. See yourself achieving your goal. Picture yourself becoming more active and enjoying it. Imagine what it would be like to eat a more varied and exciting diet.

Instead of cutting back and depriving yourself, how about experimenting with some different ways of cooking your food? You could make the process healthier by using less fat and sugar. Allow yourself to taste the food you cook, don't disguise it. Imagine you're training to become a gourmet, or a food taster for Fortnum and Mason. Eat some of your meals without ketchup, mayonnaise or brown sauce. Tasting things bare is always an experience worth having. No wonder the Häagen-Dazs sales rocketed after those famous ads. Sometimes it's like tasting something for the first time when you find out what it's like without a coating of mustard or vinegar or soy sauce.

You will discover what you really like, and how food really tastes when you're hungry. You're starting from scratch and re-educating your taste buds. You'll find, when you begin eating this way, that you won't be able to eat so fast and you will feel fuller when you've eaten less than usual.

Always be sure that the food you eat satisfies you. Don't leave the table feeling hungry. That might feel like deprivation, and if you think you're being deprived you're likely to start resenting your change in eating habits.

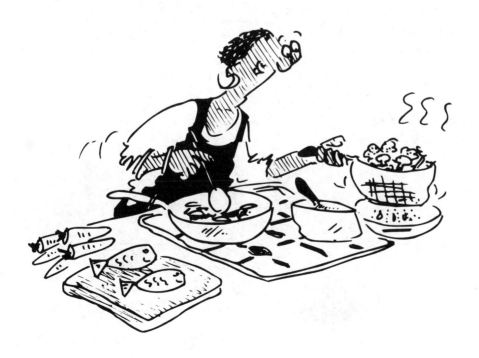

Stress...

There are two ways of dealing with stress, Quick Fixes and Relaxation.

Quick Fixes

Alcohol. A depressant. Expensive, smelly and damaging to health.

Smoking. May feel that it relaxes you but it is actually a stimulant. Expensive, smelly and damaging to health.

Caffeine. The stimulant in the three most popular drinks (apart from alcohol) world-wide: cola, coffee & tea. It won't relax you but it's not quite as disastrous health-wise as smoking and alcohol.

Overeating and undereating. Has no effect on stress other than to add to it by causing weight gain or illness.

Overwork. Has a short-term distracting effect but increases stress in the long run.

Other drugs. Expensive and may be damaging to health and relationships.

None of these will cure stress. All of them will take your mind off it briefly. In the long term they actually increase the pressure and some of them will also make you ill.

Take a moment to ask yourself:

- *What situations do you find stressful in terms of the hassles, bugs and glitches that get to you on a daily basis?*

- *How does this stress make you feel? Do you get hot, cold, anxious, cross, aroused, angry, depressed, unconscious?*

- *How do you respond to feeling this way? Do you overeat, drink, smoke, take drugs, take it out on someone, store it up inside, undereat or overwork?*

- *How might you respond differently under conditions that normally wind you up?*

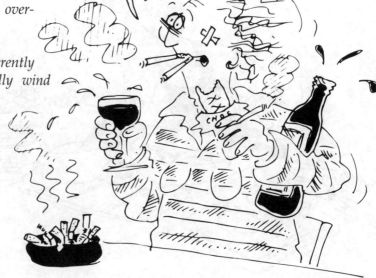

168

...And Relaxation

I know I keep going on about cars. But I've noticed over the years that a lot of my clients take much better care of their vehicles than they do of themselves. And I can't think of anyone (even me) who believes their car will run perfectly if they just put oil, petrol and water into it regularly. We know there are times when a car needs a complete service.

The rapid pace of modern life means that we don't pay much attention to our own need to take a break and give ourselves an overhaul except when we take a holiday once in a while. And holidays don't always mean rest and recreation for body and mind. They can just as easily mean a week or two of no-holds-barred eating and drinking accompanied by extreme over-exercising or extreme under-exercising. The result is a return to work feeling mentally and physically worse than before.

So far I've been talking about the minimum care you need to give your mind and body by eating sensibly and exercising regularly and being kind to yourself. But, you can do better than that. What is all the stress in your life telling you? It's telling you that you need to practise the art of relaxation and learn to let all the tension go.

You have been learning to service your body and mind by eating sensibly, by exercising and by being kind to yourself. You're ready now to acquire the wonderful habit of relaxation which renews, regenerates and helps you cope with stress. Relaxation calms you down, gives you endless energy and allows you to free yourself from external pressures. It gives you time to daydream and renew your focus on becoming slimmer, fitter and healthier.

There's no time like the present so why not pause, right now, and take a very deep breath, in through your nose and slowly breathing out through your nose again. How does that make you feel?

The act of taking a deep breath is the easiest and one of the most effective ways to relax. It's one of the reasons why a lot of people smoke – that's the only time they take a real deep breath. It's just a pity it's also highly toxic. Breathe deeply more often, especially when you are starting to feel stressed, angry or worried. My Mum used to say: *'Take a deep breath and count to ten.'* I wish I'd taken more notice of her at the time.

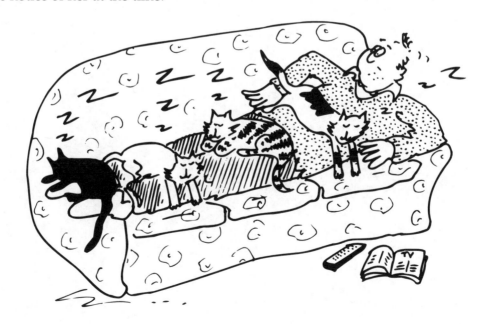

Control Yourself

This exercise is a non-violent, politically correct weapon that you can use at any time in the future to combat stress. You can use it in mixed company, at work, at home, and in the pub. This is what you do:

- When you get into the kind of situation that used to cause you stress, as soon as you feel the first physical signs of that tension, start breathing more deeply than normal. Slowly inhale the air, then release it gradually.

- If you're sitting down, stand up; it's harder to feel powerful if you're not on your feet. Plant your feet flat on the floor, roughly shoulder width apart. Ground yourself, by imagining you are a strong tree, deeply rooted in the earth. You have long, powerful roots and you can survive a hurricane.

- Imagine that all your strength comes from a point on your body about two inches below your navel. This is your centre of energy. Focus on it while you concentrate on breathing deeply and feeling how firmly you are rooted in the ground. Let the energy that comes from this point below your navel flood through your body as you feel stronger and more confident. Hold on to that feeling.

- Now think of something that is causing you to feel stress, a person or an event. And imagine yourself growing stronger while the person or the situation that upsets you shrinks rapidly to gnome size. As the cause of your anxiety gets smaller, you find yourself looking down at him or her, or it. It's hard to feel nervous, or even angry with something you could easily trample underfoot. In fact, if you've got time to plan, you might want to wear your Doc Martens for this one.

You can practise this exercise as many times as you like, and the more you run it through, the easier your brain will find it to handle that particular situation.

Strong Like Bull
with thanks to Michael Breen

Stress

Stress can knock you completely off track when you're trying to achieve something, whether it's losing weight or passing an exam. But different things are stressful for different people. It's your response that matters, not the event itself. Take holidays, for example. We're all told, particularly by travel companies, that it's good for us to take a break. But you are more likely to become ill on holiday than at any other time. Not surprising really, when you consider that holidays involve abandoning familiar routines, food, faces and climates.

Stress is a very recent idea. A hundred years ago it was just called Life. But now it's something you suffer from, like a disease. Most people get it regularly, like flu, and I suppose you can argue that we are having to cope with faster living than ever before – fast food, fast communication, fast transportation (apart from traffic jams), all in the name of convenience. Whether all this stuff makes our life more comfortable or just gives us more to worry about doesn't matter. It's our response that makes the difference between coping and collapsing under the strain.

Does it seem unfair to you that there are some people who don't seem to get stressed at all? People who even thrive on it. How do they do that? How are they managing to cope, produce great performances and sail through stormy situations? Perhaps they realise, as you are about to, that no one out there has the power to control your feelings or to make you think, behave, or act in any way other than the way you choose.

It's not the traffic jam that's putting your blood pressure up, it's your response to it. And it's probably an automatic response, just like many of your old eating habits. And if you can change your eating habits, you can also change your response to situations that make you tense.

Constructive responses involve changing your state to one of calm resourcefulness or exhilaration. And learning to use some of the many relaxation techniques is probably the best way of doing this.

Destructive responses are the quick fixes which involve drowning bad feelings rather than dealing with them. And, as you may know, quick fixes often involve food and other addictive substances.

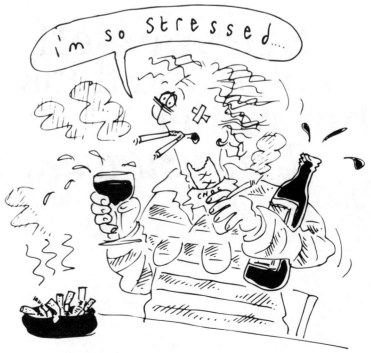

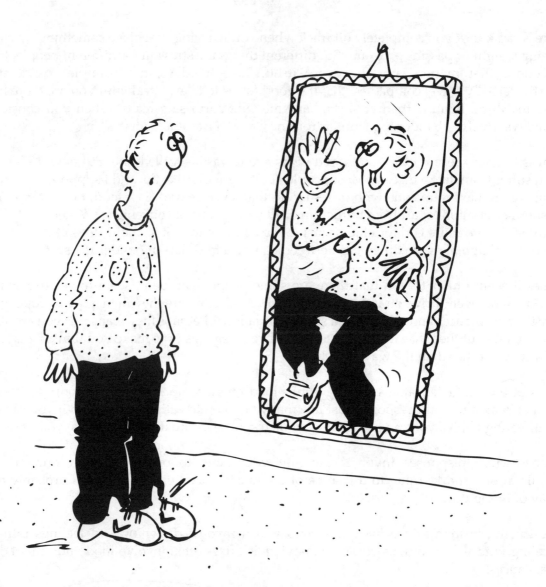

See yourself
not as you think you are,
but rather
how you want to be.

Next Week's Diary

In your own Food Diary, keep writing down:

- What you are eating and drinking.

- Where you are on the **Hunger Scale**.

- Patterns. As you identify and challenge superficial ones, you may start to see, beneath the surface, more possibilities for change than you could ever have noticed before.

- Your daily **Outcome** and whether or not you achieved it.

- When you're triggered to eat by anything other than hunger – do something else and make a note of when you succeed – and when you don't.

- How much sugar you've cut back on.

- How much water you are drinking.

- *Think Before You Eat*. This will become a life strategy and eventually your subconscious will run it for you.

- Keep a note of how much more fruit and vegetables you are eating, and watch out for the nuts and seeds as well.

- *Fill in the* **Food Cake** *until you seem to be getting naturally close to a balanced diet that feels right for your size and lifestyle. Notice the foods you're missing out on, find out why and start to identify some substitutes.*

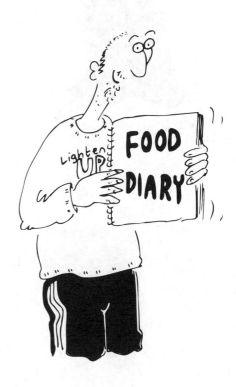

Oh, I'm so inadequate –
and I *love* myself!

Meg Ryan, actress.

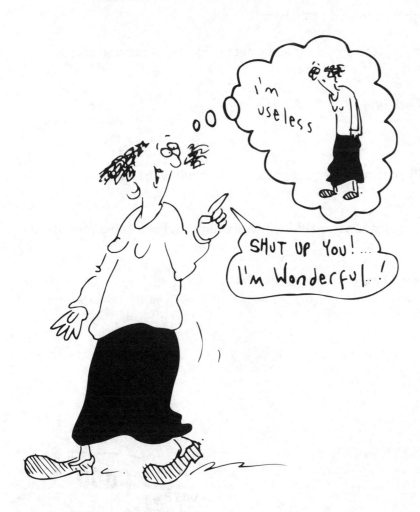

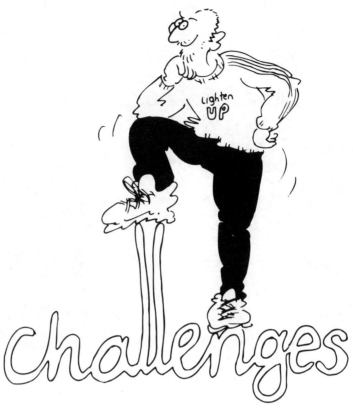

➠ Ask yourself better questions.

➠ Keep filling up your **Fat Jar**.

➠ Try a new form of exercise. There are plenty you can do by yourself, like cycling, running up and down stairs, swimming or working out to videos. And the classes and clubs you can join are almost unlimited: aerobics, Tai Chi, line dancing, gymnastics or perhaps a martial art to help keep the family in order.

➠ Use the Knife and Fork Rule.

➠ Remove the serving dishes from the table.

➠ Respond to setbacks differently as you move forwards in the right direction.

➠ Make your cooking as healthy as possible and include more nuts and seeds where you can.

➠ If you eat out, or have a takeaway, run the *Think Before You Eat* strategy first.

➠ Use conscious relaxation as a response to stress.

➠ Be your own best friend for another week. At least. If you find yourself getting attached, feel free to stay together for life.

➠ Look out for stressful situations when you can use the Control exercise.

➠ Now go back and double check that you've done all the exercises.

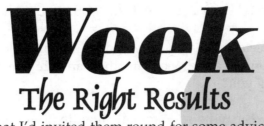

Week
The Right Results

Mo and Lisa didn't know that I'd invited them round for some advice. I'd finally invested in a new PC but it came with some flashy software that I really couldn't cope with. Both the girls were a lot more up-to-date with that sort of thing than me. We were sitting round the kitchen table with a cup of tea when Mo caught sight of the pile of boxes in the corner and said, 'You finally did it! About time too. Now I suppose it's going to take you another five years to learn this version of Windows, right?'

'That's where you come in. I want you to get me started.'

They looked at each other. Lisa said, 'I knew it wasn't just the pleasure of our company you wanted. What made you decide to upgrade, anyway?'

'There were loads of things I couldn't do on my old system,' I admitted. 'The trouble is, this new stuff is so amazing I can't do *anything* with it!'

Mo laughed, 'So the tables are turned, are they? You are always telling us that if we always do what we've always done, we'll always get what we've always got. And now you're realising that you need to make some changes as well. You may be thin and fit but you can't use *Office '97* yet.'

'I'm paying you a compliment; you two are much more *au fait* with computers than me,' I said.

'Au fat is what I feel at the moment,' said Lisa. I couldn't tell whether she was going through an ever-so-slightly-plumper than her usual skinny phase because she was wearing so many clothes. 'Honestly,' she said, 'I started another diet last week and I've broken it already. Why haven't I got any willpower, common sense or self-respect?'

'Because you keep asking yourself negative questions.' I told her. 'You won't achieve anything until you start asking yourself some more useful questions.'

'Like what?'

'Like *"How can I start to enjoy taking more exercise?"*'

'Or "Is the corner shop still open so I can nip out for a Mars Bar?"' said Mo helpfully.

I persevered. 'It's new software for your brain, Lisa. You've been running the old program so long they must be virtually hard-wired in. Come on, you can do it. Install some new ideas; ask yourself some better questions. If I can cope with a new computer, you can cope with some positive thinking.'

Lisa looked sceptical. 'That remains to be seen,' she said.

I tried to encourage her, 'Have some faith in yourself, you can do it.'

She smiled. 'Oh, I know I can stay slim – with a bit of effort. I'm not sure that you'll ever get to grips with that new PC though!'

Last Week's Food Diary And Challenges

❖ I wonder how complete and evenly balanced your **Food Cake** is looking now. Do you still have more filled in on some sections than others and are you putting much outside the circle? What is it telling you?

❖ *Think Before You Eat* may be so automatic now that you aren't actually thinking about Thinking Before You Eat any more. If you're still putting conscious effort into it, just keep going until you get there.

❖ Are new patterns still emerging? Or do you think you know your eating patterns pretty well by now?

❖ How well are the **Outcomes working** for you? Have you noticed that setting **Outcomes** is a very powerful way of focusing on achievement?

❖ Do you know now what triggers you to eat?

❖ If you took up some new forms of exercise, are you enjoying them – or did you decide the old ones weren't so bad after all?

❖ The Knife and Fork Rule may sound small, but it has a big effect.

❖ Do you ask yourself more constructive, positive questions now?

❖ Have you managed to add at least a few glasses of water to your daily intake?

❖ How did you like being your own best friend?

❖ Keep that **Fat Jar** filling up.

❖ When you're going through all this in your head, make sure you are asking yourself good quality questions about it all. Saying to yourself, *'Why am I still not drinking enough water?'* is really unhelpful. *'How can I help myself remember to drink more water?'* would be a lot more motivational.

How Are You Doing?

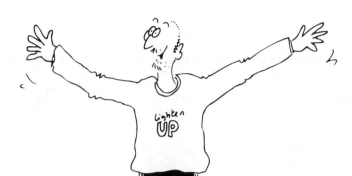

Out of all the memory joggers on the opposite page, I'm wondering which ones give you most pause for thought now. Maybe there are some ideas I've introduced that you've programmed into your brain so that you can't imagine doing things any other way. Maybe there are some techniques that you've dismissed already. If that's the case, fair enough. But, do yourself a favour – try them out again in a few weeks, just in case.

How is your **Food Cake** looking to you now? Once you decided what size cake you needed, was it easy to get enough good things in? Is it balanced? Are you leaving too many empty spaces or putting lots of extras outside the circle? Are you eating more fruit and vegetables?

Now you have all the basics, you have to decide what to concentrate on and where to put your energy. Whatever you do, **Think Before You Eat** and the **Hunger Scale** are two of the most vital pieces of brain software. These are ones I would advise you to keep going with until they become totally automatic because they are both techniques that naturally thin people tend to use.

By now you have probably learned quite a lot about your personal eating style and you will be getting to know the feelings you associate with your various eating patterns. Have you decided to dispense with any of them? And, if so, how easy did you find that?

You've done so well to get to this stage of the *Lighten Up* programme and I really hope that you've had as much fun with it as we do in the eight-week evening classes that I run. I know that reading a book on your own isn't the same as being in a group, and that's why I've suggested in some chapters that you might like to run through some of the exercises with a friend.

On the other hand, some of the *Lighten Up* ideas can be done just as easily, if not more easily, by yourself. **Outcomes** is one of them. Did you find that was a helpful way of setting up your day?

And what about all the other ideas? Have you found a form of exercise that makes you happy and fits easily into your daily life? Have you tried something new? Take the knife and fork rule, for example. It's a simple little idea that may have seemed strange and difficult at first, but it's surprising how quickly you become used to pausing for thirty seconds or so between bites and really enjoying your food.

Alcohol...

Reasons for Drinking: *There's only one. To enjoy it. And that means taking it slowly and savouring every sip.*

- Drink in moderation.

- Drink water with it and don't drink on an empty stomach.

- If you take a drink, take it slowly. Wine with a meal shouldn't be used just to wash down the food.

- Never use it to quench thirst. It's a diuretic.

- If you're drinking spirits, ask yourself if you might substitute wine or beer.

- Be aware of how alcohol is making you feel and how much you have drunk.

- Drink at your own pace, unless it's faster than everybody else's.

- The fewer chemicals in your chosen drink, the less harm it will do to you. Read the labels.

- If you drink spirits at home, think small pub measures.

- Spend more on buying high quality and drink less of it.

...In Moderation

By now you should be clear on the need to cut down or cut out refined sugar from your diet. However, there is another substance that many people are drawn to because it makes them feel even better than sugar. It has other attractions too, it's a very social activity and it can be addictive.

Alcohol is a drug, but it's also the highest-calorie quick fix for stress, apart from overeating. It's fast becoming our third major health hazard in the UK after heart disease and cancer. There are seventy calories in a glass of wine, it doesn't add anything to your diet nutritionally and it can even cause vitamin deficiencies.

Like sugar, it's absorbed into the bloodstream very quickly. If you drink alcohol that has sugar in it, you are subjecting your body to a double harmful dose. Drinking alcohol can seriously damage your health and it only takes around four units a day, over a period of time, to cause liver damage in an average size person.

Another problem with alcohol is that, being a depressant, it often stops you noticing how much you're eating. And drinking with food isn't a good idea anyway because fluid dilutes the digestive enzymes, and the longer food sloshes around in the stomach the harder it is to digest.

A study at Maastricht University in the Netherlands found that drinking before and during meals made people eat more quickly and scoff bigger portions. It can take out your inhibitions and encourage you to eat more.

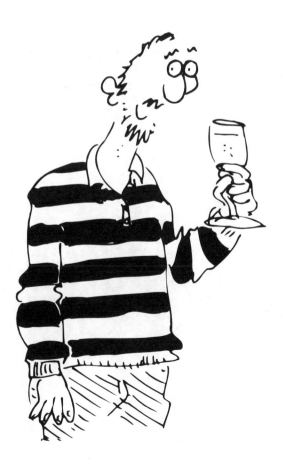

You Are What You Eat...

The basic guidelines for being slimmer, fitter, healthier, more energetic and living longer are:

- Increase your unrefined carbohydrate intake, vary it as much as you can by including brown rice, pasta, couscous, bulgur, buckwheat, keniou, millet, potatoes, carrots and parsnips.

- Cut down on refined sugars, salt and caffeine. They play havoc with our bodies, confusing and interrupting the natural running order.

- Drink lots of fresh water (I may have mentioned this before).

- Give yourself time and space to eat and enjoy your meals.

- Whenever possible, choose fresh foods with no additives, preservatives, E numbers or added sugar and eat some of them raw. Don't overcook your veggies because that destroys some of the nutritional value.

- Eat less red meat and deep fried food.

- As I've said about a million times already, be creative, try different grains, fruits and vegetables and experiment with new recipes.

- Be curious about ingredients. Read labels, not to count the calories, just to check what you're putting inside you. If you don't know what it is, the chances are it's not good for you, so don't eat it.

- Eat more nuts and seeds. They are full of energy, protein, oils, vitamins and minerals.

- Look for balance. As you start to respect your body more, give it more of the foods it really wants and listen to the response. Let your body tell you when it's hungry and when it's full.

- Don't eat something just because it's healthy. Make gradual changes and enjoy what you eat.

...*So Eat What You Are*

We are omnivores, which means that, like pigs, we'll eat any old rubbish that's lying around and generally survive on it. In fact, it's probably the key to our survival. If our diet was as limited as the giant panda or even the koala, it's unlikely that we'd have populated most of the planet and multiplied at the rate we did.

If you take a strictly herbivorous animal and feed it meat, there's a good chance that something bad may happen to it, which is one of the theories about mad cow disease. Human beings are more resilient, however. We can eat anything from whale blubber to bugs and get by. But, however tolerant our bodies are, there is some evidence that they do better on fresh, natural foods.

Unfortunately, because we have learned to eat for reasons other than hunger, we have formed strong associations with sugary, salty foods that are easy to eat when we aren't hungry at all. A lot of these snacks are full of chemicals (which our bodies have only had a few years of learning to tolerate) as well as sugar, fat and salt. Perhaps the genetically modified human beings of the future will do very well on the food, water and air that is toxic to us right now. But, for the moment, we are still fairly primitive organisms as far as food is concerned and we flourish on a fairly primitive diet.

Nutrition is still a young science in the Western World, but it is fast establishing links between diet and disease. Minor changes in your eating habits can lead to major changes in your size, shape and state of health.

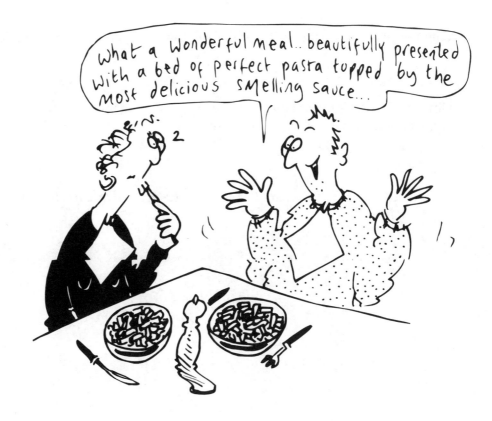

Relaxation

Relaxation is the only sure-fire, long-term method of coping with stress. It's cheap, it's not anti-social and it doesn't damage your health.

It sounds obvious. So why are dysfunctional eating and chemicals still such popular stress busters?

There is one major problem with relaxation. It works only when it's personalised and that takes time and energy and effort. Before you can make it work for you, you have to get to know yourself better.

- Identify your personal pressure points, like particular people or events.

- Look at the next pages for some ideas on relaxation.

- Practise them until they become automatic responses.

- Take a moment to make a quick list of the things which put pressure on you every day. Your 'daily hassles'. We aren't talking about big stuff like Death, Marriage and Moving House. Just the bugs and glitches that get to you on a daily (or weekly) basis.

- Think of five of your favourites and write them down in your notebook.

- How are you dealing with these problems at the moment? Try and come up with more than two techniques that you habitually use.

If you've included any of the quick fixes (like alcohol), be prepared to start eliminating them over the next few weeks or months.

The Truth Is Out There

It's everywhere, it's an epidemic and if you haven't got it, you obviously haven't lived.

Stress is credited with causing almost as much death and despair as war. At one time or another it's been blamed for just about every fashionable ailment from migraine to cancer. The interesting thing is that it's not actually *out there* at all. It's just a feeling we mix ourselves with our own personal chemicals. We can say it's a response to the new job, the new baby, the new relationship, or even the old job, the teenager and the divorce. But the truth is that an event that's stressful for one person will be exciting and challenging for another.

Stress isn't something you catch from someone else and it's not something other people do to you. There aren't even any universally stressful situations. If there were, there wouldn't be surgeons, ambulance drivers and mercenary soldiers.

There is no stress out there, not one bit. You've manufactured it personally, tailored to your own personal tastes. You make the decisions about what you want to be stressful, whether it's losing your car keys, missing your train, overworking, boredom, or coping with a toddler. Hundreds of times a day we activate our own personal stress response. Our brains start buzzing and breathing becomes faster as we get tense and tight. If this response becomes habitual, we start to experience negative emotions like anger, sadness, low self-esteem and anxiety.

But we are also creatures of comfort, so we need a break and we look for some pleasure to ease the pain. So, we reach for the quick fixes: eating, smoking, drinking and whatever other chemicals are acceptable and affordable to us. The sadly predictable result is short-term relief followed by a long-term intensification of the stress symptoms. Even more sadly, although the stress doesn't actually exist, our reaction to it often causes very real health problems and a poor quality of life.

The Answer isn't out there either.

Fortunately, we are all born with the antidote to the problem as well as the cause. It's a simple matter of reversing our normal process and relaxing the mind while exercising the body. This takes a little practice, and of course a decision to change. But that's all.

As your body becomes fitter and stronger, your mind will learn to let go and relax.

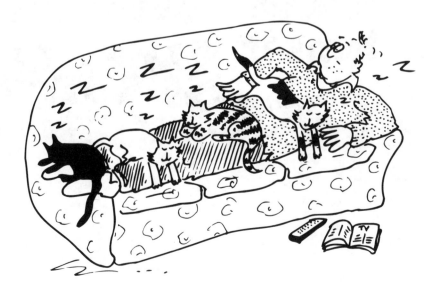

Peaceful Mind

For the man who has conquered his mind, it is his greatest friend;
6ut for the
man who fails to do so,
his mind
will 6e his greatest enemy.
Sri Krishna

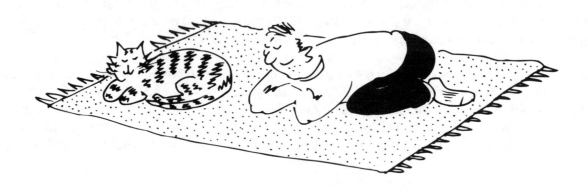

One who overcomes
others has force;
one who overcomes
himself is strong.
Taoist poem

Relaxed Body

Adjust Your Surroundings

Find a calm place. It doesn't even have to be a place. It could be when you're walking, taking a bath or having a massage. Furnish your mind like a sanctuary, a warm, sandy beach, a cosy fireside, a quiet forest clearing, or a moonlit verandah on a hot night. Allow harmony, peace, quiet voices. Choose a positive idea and have it to hand. Play music in your head and tell yourself a story.

Physical Activity

Exercise works for a lot of people because it uses up stress hormones in a natural way, restoring the body to a healthy balance. Dancing, gardening, jogging or walking the dog, to name but a few.

Mirroring Relaxation

This is kangaroo care for grown-ups. Tune into another creature's ability to relax. Watch the fish, stroke the cat, go horse riding. Human beings behave like harmless parasites with certain animals. We absorb their calm and steady breathing and their inability to worry.

But be careful. It can work in reverse. Nervous animals and stressed, aggressive people transmit negative energy and raise your blood pressure if you get close to them.

Visualisation

Take a moment to yourself, choose a feeling that will make you feel good and go to the part of your mind that stores that feeling. Relive the experience. See yourself in the future where you will be feeling the same feeling and when it will benefit you most. Let your imagination fill in the gaps. The technical name for this technique is daydreaming.

Massage

Massage, reflexology and aromatherapy are all external interventions which work through more than one sense at a time. Touch and smell together can be powerful relaxants.

Find relaxers that work for you and indulge, often.

Chilling Out

- Find a quiet place where you can sit without being disturbed for ten to twenty minutes.

- Sit comfortably, with your back straight, facing forward, and both feet flat on the floor. Turn the lighting down or off.

- Focus on your breathing as you notice the gentle rise and fall of your chest. Follow your breath in through your nose, right into your body and back out through your nose.

- Follow your breath now with a little more concentration. Be aware of the air streaming in through your nostrils and filling your lungs. Imagine you can see the air being drawn down deeper into your body, filling it with life.

- Keep your breathing at the front of your mind so that you become aware of it without thinking about it.

- If any thoughts creep into your head, acknowledge them and let them go. You might wonder why certain things come into your mind and you might feel obliged to go with a thought. Push it away. Imagine putting all those thoughts into the bin or down the waste disposal unit and bring your attention back to your breath.

- Begin to count your breaths at the end of every outward breath. Hear yourself saying the number.

- If you lose your place or forget the number it doesn't matter. Just start again at the beginning. The counting is simply to focus your attention on your breathing.

- You might find that some days your mind is more active than others, but just expect whatever you experience and notice the deep relaxation and peace you feel.

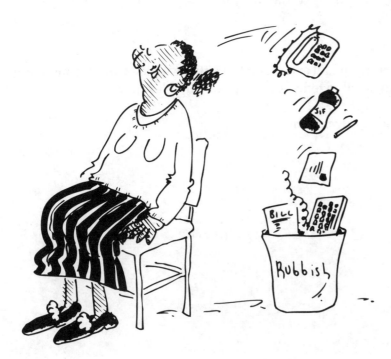

188

The Technique

There are lots of ways to cope with the negative side effects of stress. And some of them will even enable you to live a stress-free life.

The **Chilling Out** technique is one of these and, by practising it every day, you will learn to be more positive as you get better and better at coping with stressful situations. You will also become more relaxed and your general health and wellbeing will improve.

Chilling Out teaches your brain to do exactly the opposite of what it does when you become stressed. It teaches greater control of your thoughts and profound levels of rest. Imagine how good you feel when you stop worrying about things you can't control.

Practising this technique trains your mind to focus on just one thing at a time. Which is not something we naturally do. Your ability to relax at will increases as you teach yourself how to have greater control over your thoughts and dissolve stress and tension.

This exercise is often met with resistance, and the resistance comes from ourselves. Our minds are normally active and that's what they're used to. It's the mental status quo. The **Chilling Out** technique teaches the mind to behave counter-intuitively, so it's bound to take a little while.

Everybody wants instant results, which is why the quick fix remedies for any discomfort are so popular. **Chilling Out** is not a quick fix remedy. If you want it to work for you, you need to put it in the same place as your new commitment to a more active lifestyle. It's something you will do regularly, until it becomes second nature to you. And you'll do it because you want to permanently feel relaxed and calm.

It's such a simple, straightforward way of relaxing that you might ask yourself how it could possibly be so effective. The answer is to practise it and see. All you need to do is give yourself ten minutes morning and evening. If you like it, you can gradually increase this to twenty minutes over the next few weeks.

It is better to practise this routine before you eat, but it is totally compatible with exercise. In fact, some people get the same result through walking or some other form of exercise. But you won't know if this technique will be a regular habit for you until you give it a fair trial. And, even if it's not going to be part of your daily life, it's well worth learning the breathing technique for use in stressful situations. Whenever you find yourself under pressure, just take a moment to follow your breath and let yourself relax as you increase your control.

189

Change Reaction

The techniques and ideas I've put into this book are aimed at teaching you to use your mind and body in the most powerful and advantageous ways. With your desire and your ability to take action by using the exercises that are right for you, you can be slimmer forever.

Some people are born with advantages: a powerful, healthy physique, money, a supportive family and great educational opportunities. Maybe, you might say, some people are born thin. But there are plenty of people who didn't start out with any of those advantages and they still ended up looking good, feeling good and attracting as much love and money as they wanted.

How did they do that? From what I've seen and observed, it was by making committed decisions about what they wanted and following those decisions with action for change.

This is the process:

Questions:

'Do I expect to achieve my goals?'

'Can I see myself looking like and feeling like the person I want to be?'

'Can I run that as a movie in which I'm ideally qualified for the leading role?'

If the answer to this is *'Yes'*, go on to Part Two.

If the answer is *'No'*, you have two choices:
> (1) keep working on your beliefs until you get a clear strong *'Yes'*, or,
> (2) stay as you are and like yourself that way.

Statement: *'I am getting slimmer.'*

Decision: *'I know what it takes and I'm already doing it.'*

Just Do It.

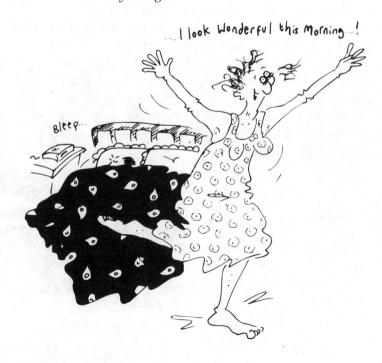

Believe It And You Are Ready To Achieve It

If you put some effort into *believing* what you want, the effort you put into *achieving* it will seem relatively easy.

Do you believe you can be slimmer?

Whether you believe you can or believe you can't, you're right. It's up to you to pull your own strings. All the effort and energy you put into being slimmer won't necessarily get you there unless you really believe it's possible. The function of your brain is to confirm what you believe. So, if you believe you're fat, stupid or you can't do something, you're right.

If I asked you: *'Is breathing good for you?'* what would your answer be? If you say: *'Yes, of course it is'*, how do you know? Well, you've experienced it, that's how you know. But what other strong beliefs do you have?

> *War is a bad thing.*

> *Exhaust fumes are damaging our environment.*

> *Life's a beach and then you fry.*

You weren't born believing in any of the those; you learned to believe them. That's how beliefs are formed. You will have plenty of references as to why you believe in something; maybe you were told by your parents, you read about it, you discussed it and now you believe it. Sometimes we hold on to beliefs built on references that are obsolete, outdated or outgrown.

Perfectly intelligent people have been known to live their lives thinking they were completely stupid, solely on the basis of random remarks their teachers made. Beliefs which are strong enough to limit our lives and make us unhappy often have flimsy foundations.

Beliefs are just rules and generalisations that we have made for ourselves. How can we ever know which ones are valid and which ones aren't? How do we know which ones to live by and which ones to abandon?

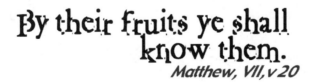

By their fruits ye shall know them.
Matthew, VII, v 20

If your beliefs serve you well, if they help you to become slimmer, richer, happier, more confident, then they are good ones to have. If your beliefs are making you unhappy, dysfunctional and fat, they probably need to be binned. Pronto.

Do You Believe You Can Be Slimmer?

Some beliefs have firmer foundations than others. If you want your positive beliefs to withstand an earthquake, you need to reinforce their foundations.

If you believe you can be slimmer, what is supporting that?

A really strong foundation for your belief in your ability to become slimmer might be built on some of these:

I'm exercising.	☐
I'm being patient.	☐
I'm being positive.	☐
I'm thinking before I eat.	☐
I'm using my **Affirmation.**	☐
I'm thinking before I buy.	☐
I'm eating a balanced diet.	☐
I'm filling in the **Food Cake**.	☐
I've slowed down my eating.	☐
I'm setting myself **Outcomes**.	☐
I'm drinking plenty of water.	☐
I'm writing down what I eat.	☐
I'm taking my **Fat-Burning Pills**.	☐
I'm eating more nutritious foods.	☐
I can refuse food if I'm not really hungry.	☐
I'm learning from everything that has happened to me.	☐

What else are you doing to support the belief that you are reaching the goal?

Attention

The greatest discovery of my generation
is that human beings can alter their lives by altering their states of mind.
William James

Whatever you pay attention to, and what you decide to think about, affects how you feel and what you do. We all move towards whatever we regularly, consistently focus on and imagine. Occasional thoughts may flit through our minds. But it's only the regular, persistent offenders that can ruin our life.

Ask yourself:

'What have I been thinking about the most, today and every day for the past week?'

'Have these thoughts been helpful, encouraging and optimistic? Or not?'

Most people think about what others think or what others are doing. True champions tend to be much more concerned with themselves and what they can control. Every thought can have two consequences: it either moves you closer to your dreams or takes you further away.

The first step towards positive change is to start thinking it's possible. Most of us don't seem to think that way and maybe that's why only 10% of people who buy a book like this read past the first chapter and less than 10% of people bother to write down their goals.

The second step towards positive change is to put positive thoughts into action. Why do so few people live the life of their dreams? Because it takes effort and action. If you don't follow up your dreams by taking action, you still won't get what you want.

Let's look at another 10% to illustrate this one. Everybody knows that in order to be slimmer, fitter and healthier we need to be physically active. Millions of people in the UK would like to be slimmer, fitter and healthier than they are – so why is it that only 10% of the population actually makes the effort to take enough exercise?

Very few people actually walk their talk. Yet, that is all they need to do.

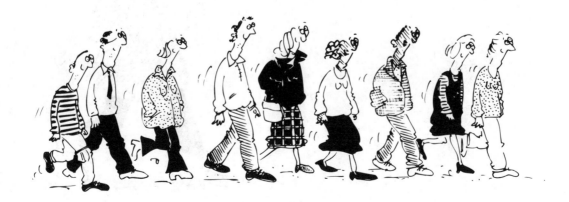

Walk Your Talk

Excellence in anything depends on how you answer these five questions:

1. Who do you think is responsible for the change you want to make?

2. How well do you know where you want to go? Check whether you can picture it, hear it and feel it in your mind – or whether it's still a little out of focus.

3. How much do you really want to be there? You need to know what it is that you'll get out of this change you have in mind. You have to be aware of the details: exactly *how* your life will be different and how *you* will feel about yourself when it happens.

4. How strongly do you believe in your ability to achieve this **Outcome** that you want? Check out the evidence supporting your belief that this is what you want.

5. Are you ready and willing to take action?

If your belief in your ability to make your changes is a still a little shaky, strengthen the foundations of that belief with some of these:

*   Exercising regularly so that it becomes an enjoyable part of your daily life.

*   Learning from your mistakes instead of blaming yourself for them.

*   Drinking more water rather than tea, coffee and soft drinks.

*   Eating a healthy, balanced diet.

*   Eating only when your body tells you that you really are hungry.

*   Checking in advance what kind of food would feel good inside you.

*   Being much nicer to yourself.

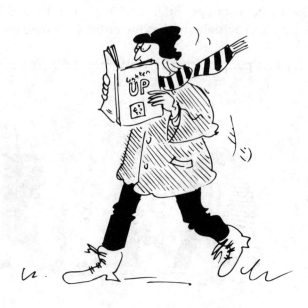

Willing And Responsible

The questions on the left aren't ones you can answer quickly. Take the time to think them through. You are looking to find out whether you are really ready to change and become slimmer, fitter and healthier than you have been before. It all depends on the strength of your belief in your ability to change and your belief in whether the change is right for you.

Some beliefs have stronger foundations than others. Once you've built the belief, you can set about reinforcing the foundations. You are probably getting slimmer and you believe that you will be a slim person in the future.

A lot of people go through life blaming others when things go wrong. We all do it sometimes. When you give responsibility for your life to others, you are depriving yourself of a precious opportunity to learn, because you can't learn from other people's mistakes as easily as you can from your own.

~~Try~~ Re-phrasing It

A lot of people will tell you they gave something their best shot, that they tried really hard, or that they persevered as long as they could. This is the language of failure. People who really want something don't use words like *must, should, ought, try,* or *persevere.* The minute you start talking to yourself in language like that you sow the seeds of doubt in your mind. Then the whole enterprise starts looking like really hard work.

So start by overhauling your vocabulary. Get rid of *'I'd like to', 'I hope'* and *'I might'*. These words just don't have the power to positively change your life or enhance it.

If you really want something, first, you've got to be willing to take all the actions required to take you there. Second, you've got to understand that you alone are responsible; responsible for doing whatever it takes to get where you want to go.

This frees you up from blaming others and allows you to focus on yourself and what you need to do to achieve your goal.

What Works For You

- Is it the **Think Before You Eat** strategy?

- Using the **Hunger Scale**?

- Eating more slowly so that you know when you're full?

- Doing something else when you're triggered to eat for reasons other than hunger?

- Becoming more active?

- Making a meal of food and separating it from other activities so that you really enjoy it?

- Drinking loads of water through the day?

- Translating failures into feedback and taking action?

- Learning from your experience about losing weight?

- Eating a wider variety of foods than before?

- Developing new strategies for coping with stress?

- Deleting some of the bad, old stress-relieving strategies (like eating)?

- Being your own best friend?

- Getting pleasure from new sources?

By the way, if you really have to do it, now might be a good time to weigh yourself.

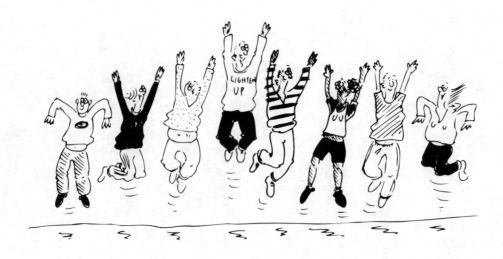

What's The Difference That Makes The Difference For You?

Do you remember what you wanted to achieve in Week One? Look back at the **Outcomes** you set for yourself in Weeks One and Two. Would you do them all over again – or are your priorities different now?

It's important to re-evaluate this because it may be that what you want has changed. Or perhaps you've already achieved it and it's time, now, to pursue your more challenging goals.

Knowing what you want is vital. Otherwise you might never get it. Worse still, you won't even know when you have got it.

Think back over the past eight weeks and review all your successes. How many things have you done that you're proud of?

Make a list of the ideas and exercises that have made the difference for you.

- *What's worked and what have you done to get to this point?*

- *What do you want now and for the future?*

- *What's your plan for getting what you want?*

- *What is it precisely that you need to do now to get exactly what you want?*

Life is not
the way it's supposed
to be,
it's the way it is.
The way you cope with it
is what makes the difference.

— Virginia Satir

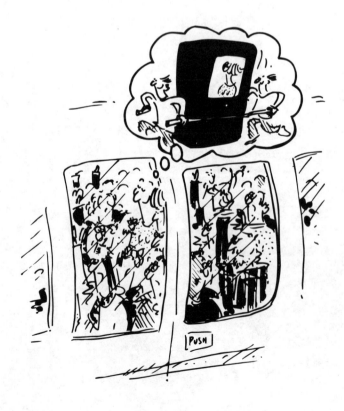

Diary For Life

Keep your **Food Diary**, writing down what you eat and drink for the next four weeks. Keep it in your own format and record what seems important to you. After four weeks I'm confident that most of you will continue with it because the reasons for writing it will become very clear when you're doing it for yourself – rather than because I'm telling you to. Personally, I find that keeping a diary keeps me on track. Although I do censor it.

Censorship

Just as I'm always telling you to give yourself positive messages, I'm also suggesting that you write positive things in the diary as well. There are lots of reasons for keeping a diary but one of the most important ones is to make sure that the software you run in your own brain is positive, constructive and helpful.

I'm not saying, *'Don't write down the negative stuff'*. Of course, you'll have lapses and bad days, and you need to make a note of them so that you can look back a couple of weeks later and see how insignificant they were. That's very encouraging.

Nevertheless, the really important thing is to write down the good stuff so that you really know what's working and you can congratulate yourself and take heart from it. Write down what you've learned from the things that have gone wrong – much more important than recording the actual disasters. Write down the things you've achieved, how you've felt about them and the progress you are making towards your goal. When you get there, by the way, you may have to set a whole new **Outcome**. Positive changes never let you rest. Once you're hooked on change you'll find you have to keep going. It's an addiction of the best kind.

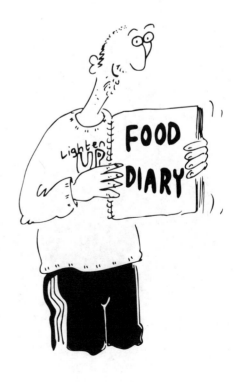

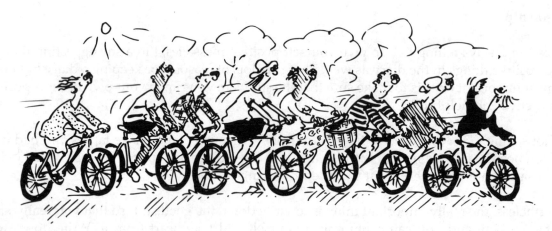

The past is over, the future's not here yet,
but this moment, right now, is a gift,
that's why it's called the present.
                    Sign over a bar in San Antonio.

➠ This week you get all the exercises in the whole book as your **Challenges**. Of course you can cherry pick, but always give the ones that didn't work first time a second chance.

➠ Relax more as you respond to stress differently. Experiment with the relaxation techniques I've suggested and research some more of your own until you find the ones that work for you.

➠ Continue to feel good for no good reason. I always say that – but, come to think of it, any reason to feel good is a good reason, isn't it?

➠ Remember the **Hunger Scale**? By now you may be clocking where you are on that automatically. If not, keep going with it consciously until it becomes second nature.

➠ Keep going with **Think Before You Eat** until it's programmed in. It's like a shield you can carry for the rest of your life that will protect you from eating the wrong things.

➠ Daydream on. The **Pink Elephant** should be a neon sign by now – with your New You picture glowing alongside it. This is the fun bit. Whenever you get disheartened, or you can't cope with working out your **Hunger Scale**, try a bit of **Daydreaming With Intent**. Catching a glimpse of the Future You that you really want to be is very energising.

➠ Use the **Chilling Out** technique at every opportunity.

➠ Make sure you get plenty of health food for your mind as well as your body.

➠ Design yourself a plan of action for the next month.

➠ Make a contract with yourself to follow the plan.

➠ Follow the **Success Formula**.

Good Luck.

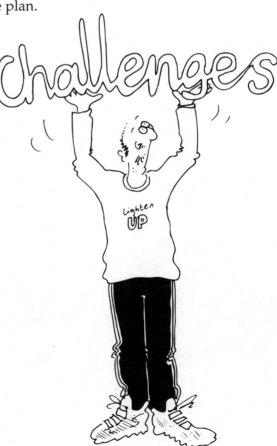

Ideas
And
Recipes

Top Tips

- Invest in a water filter. It dramatically improves the quality and taste of tap water, it's cheaper than bottled water and saves carrying so much back from the supermarket.

- Read food labels carefully; if an ingredient has a scientific name, it probably has E numbers.

- Freeze left-over wine in an ice cube tray. Then use a cube or two in sauce for flavour.

- Have some cooked rice in the freezer for times when you are late home or in a hurry.

- Keep a complete emergency meal in the freezer or store cupboard.

- Freeze left-over vegetables for soup.

- Freeze sliced bread and put it straight in the toaster. It's much nicer when it's very fresh.

- Whip up cottage cheese as an alternative to mayonnaise.

- Wrap fish or skinless chicken in greaseproof paper with wine or fruit juice and bake.

- Sprinkle fresh herbs and black pepper on your vegetables instead of butter.

- Sauté vegetables in fat-free stock.

- For a special meal, try dry pan-fried fresh tuna. It's wonderful.

- Venison, partridge and rabbit are very low in fat for the rich or adventurous.

- Crisp up stale rice cakes or crackers in a hot oven for five minutes.

- Keep dried fruit for when you want something very sweet.

- Try balsamic vinegar or lemon juice on your salad instead of dressing.

- Next time you order a pizza, ask for a thin wholemeal base with half or no cheese.

Food Cupboard Basics

If your cupboard is well stocked, you'll be less likely to succumb to temptation, have a fit of the munchies and resort to the corner-shop for high-fat microwave snacks.

Long grain brown rice
Wild rice
Whole wheat pasta
Whole wheat noodles or buckwheat
Porridge oats
Red lentils (no need to soak)
Kidney beans (tinned or dried)
Any other beans or lentils

Olive oil
Garlic (tube or fresh)
Soy sauce
Tomato puree (tube and tins)
Balsamic vinegar
Wine vinegar
Mustard
Vegetable stock cubes
Marmite

Tins of salmon and tuna (in brine or water)
Chick peas

Basil (dried or frozen, but best fresh)
Marjoram
Sage
Ginger
Curry powder or paste
Italian mixed herbs
Low sodium salt
Black pepper
Cinnamon

Dried fruit
Fresh fruit

Clues For Reading Labels

If it has a scientific name, it's usually man-made and has an E number.

If you don't recognise the names, they are probably not natural.

Nutritional value is measured in
> Protein
> Fat
> Carbohydrates (simple and complex)
> Minerals and vitamins

If a label doesn't have calorific values on it, remember that any fat has 9 calories per gram but protein and carbohydrate only have 4 calories per gram.

If an item is really cheap it's almost certainly composed largely of chemicals and if you look at the label, the name of the product (pizza, bread) may be the only thing you may recognise.

Rather than looking for perfection, look for balance and a variety of foods from different food groups.

Look to buy as many natural fresh products as possible. See packaged food and tinned food as dead food, and natural foods as life foods – foods that will give you life energy, and vitality.

All Day Breakfast

Sliced banana with rolled oats, orange juice and plain low fat yoghurt.

Fresh fruit salad with fromage frais.

Sesame Ryvita topped with cottage cheese and sliced nectarine.

Steamed banana on wholemeal toast.

Grilled grapefruit sprinkled with soft brown sugar.

Weetabix with freshly squeezed orange juice and raspberries.

Grated apple with fruit muesli and soya milk.

Lean trimmed grilled bacon on wholemeal toast.

Potato waffles with poached egg and grilled tomatoes.

Mushroom and black pepper omelette.

Scrambled eggs with smoked salmon.

Baked beans on wholemeal muffins.

Grilled cottage cheese and Worcester sauce on crumpets.

Tomatoes on toast with grated melted Edam.

Grilled kippers with tinned plum tomatoes.

Porridge cooked with dates and grated pear.

Chocolate porridge made with cocoa and brown sugar.

Sensational Snacks

Home-made Popcorn With Mixed Fruit
Sprinkle the mixed dried fruit over the fresh popcorn with a little cinnamon. Keep in an airtight container.

Porridge With Apple and Dates
Chop a few dates and an eating apple. Add to the oats and water with a dash of milk and a sprinkle of cinnamon. Cook until the apples are soft.

Apple and Pear Chips
Thinly slice the fruit. Cook in a hot oven on greaseproof paper until crisp. Be careful not to overcook.

Orange French Eggie Bread
Whip egg with the juice of half an orange and half a teaspoon of soft brown sugar. Heat the frying pan with a spray of oil. Soak a slice of wholemeal bread in the mixture then cook on both sides. Another good version is lemon juice and honey.

Freshly Squeezed OJ Ice Lollies
Make your own or go to Marks & Spencer.

Grated Apple and Yoghurt
Add to the apple and low fat plain yoghurt a tablespoon of muesli or oats with a dash of orange juice.

Baked Sweet Potato
Cook in a hot oven until soft. Eat hot or cold.

Vegetable Sticks with Hoummus or Smoked Salmon Dip
For a low fat hoummus, blend tinned or soaked chick peas with 1 teaspoon of garlic and 2 teaspoons of tahini. To make the smoked salmon dip, blend a small tub of cottage cheese, a teaspoon of tomato puree, a dash of anchovy paste or pâté with 50g of smoked salmon. Try dipping raw mushrooms to make a change from carrot sticks.

Corn on the Cob
Steam or boil. Serve with sprinkle of fresh Parmesan.

Oven Chips
2 lbs potatoes,1 dessertspoon olive oil, herbs, if required.

Wash and dry the potatoes thoroughly. Leaving the peel on, cut into chunks approximately one-inch thick (chip-like shapes). Dry again in a cloth, then place in a large bowl with olive oil and a little salt. Add herbs if you like them. Toss well, spread out onto a baking tray and place in a Mark 8/230 C oven on a high shelf for about 30 minutes until golden brown and crisp. They may take slightly longer depending on your oven and the potatoes!

Yummy Roasted Vegetables

Olive oil, garlic and onion and any vegetables that you like to try. It comes out differently every time depending on the vegetables that you use. Try sweet potatoes, cauliflower, broccoli.

Just cut the vegetables into large chunks (smaller for carrots, parsnips, sweet potatoes) and place in a large bowl with the minimum amount of olive oil to coat them all. You won't need too much. Roast on a baking tray on a high shelf of an 180 C oven for approximately 40 minutes. Make regular checks as progress will depend on which vegetables you have used. Add herbs if you like – sprigs of rosemary give a wonderful flavour. Serve as is or with couscous, pasta or rice. Makes a wonderful sandwich filling when cold.

Jacket Potatoes with:

Curried cottage cheese and grapes

Ratatouille and lean chicken breast

Tuna fish and mixed beans in a chilli sauce

Tofu diced tomato with a miso paste sauce

Prawn, grated cucumber, fromage frais, lemon juice and mayonnaise

Cold baked beans and cottage cheese

Sliced hard-boiled eggs, lean bacon and tomato sauce

Smoked trout and lime juice

Dry stir-fry onion, mushrooms, peppers, sweetcorn and turkey

Steamed spinach and poached egg

Leeks in tomato sauce and fresh parmesan

Stir fry spring onion, sliced mange tout, baby corn heads, lean pork, grated ginger and soy sauce

Great Ideas For Rolls, Pitta Bread, Baguettes, Bagels, etc.

Smoked salmon, low fat cream cheese, chives and lemon.

Ham and slices of melon.

Tuna, spring onion and tomato puree.

Avocado pear and prawns.

Crab sticks, miso and cucumber.

Strawberries, black pepper and low fat cream cheese.
    (the pepper brings out the flavour in the fruit)

Kiwi fruit and cottage cheese.

Watercress, boiled egg and tomato.

Alfalfa sprouts and peanut butter.

Tuna, sweetcorn, fromage frais and curry paste.

Low fat hoummus and salad.

Smoked tofu, tomato chutney and cress.

Char-grilled vegetables and fresh Parmesan cheese.

Banana and strawberry yoghurt.
    (choose a thick yoghurt for spreading)

Smoked trout and cucumber.

Beetroot and grated Edam cheese.

Boxed Lunches

Taking food to work is always a great idea. It stops you making impulsive choices and ensures that you will have something good to eat exactly when you want it. Try these ideas and invent some of your own.

Tuna and Pasta Salad
1 ½ cups of cooked brown pasta
½ cup of chopped red peppers
¼ cup of sweetcorn
½ cup of chopped cucumber
½ cup of chopped baby tomatoes
¼ cup of finely chopped raw onion (optional)
small tin of tuna in brine (well drained)
sprinkle of chopped parsley
1 ½ teaspoons of soy sauce
3 tablespoons of low fat fromage frais

Mix all ingredients well.

Quorn and Rice Salad
1 cup of long grain cooked brown rice
1 cup of Quorn chunks
½ cup of cold cooked peas
½ cup of yellow or red peppers
½ cup of seedless green grapes
1 ½ teaspoons sesame oil
1 teaspoon of grated ginger
2 teaspoons of Chinese vinegar
1 tablespoon of roasted sesame seeds.

Mix all ingredients well and eat cold.

Fruit Drinks

You can use any fruit as long as it's ripe. Experiment as you come up with some smooth operators! If you want your drinks chilled, add some ice cubes.

Cool Runnings
1 banana
1 apple with skin
1 kiwi fruit
1 pear with skin
½ pint of milk or rice milk
handful of brazil nuts or any nuts
tablespoon of flaked coconut

Blend and serve.

Island in the Sun
15g coconut milk powder
300ml warm water
350g pineapple flesh
175g banana flesh
75ml pineapple juice
2 tablespoons lime juice
a little lime zest

Blend the coconut milk powder with the warm water. Set aside to cool.

Place the pineapple flesh in a food processor. Process briefly. Add the banana flesh and process until smooth. Then gradually add the pineapple juice, prepared coconut milk and lime juice.

Process briefly. Pour into tall glasses to serve and decorate with a little lime zest.

Melon and Strawberry Cooler
350g strawberries
350g melon flesh, cubed
150ml apple juice

Place the strawberries in a food processor with the melon. Process until smooth. Gradually add the apple juice and process briefly. Pour the melon and strawberry cooler into tall glasses to serve.

Soups

Carrot and Parsnip Soup
Serves 6.

Olive oil
1 large onion chopped
450g young carrots chopped
225g parsnips
1 litre of vegetable stock
1 clove of garlic, crushed
2 teaspoons ground coriander
2 tablespoons chopped fresh coriander

Heat and coat a large saucepan with olive oil. Fry the onion with the garlic until soft. Add the celery and cook for a few minutes. Add the stock, carrots and parsnips. Cover and simmer for about 15 minutes. Reduce the heat and add the ground coriander, cook for a further 2 – 3 minutes, then either blend, or mash, and reheat slowly in the saucepan adding the chopped coriander. Season to taste.
Serve with a swirl of plain yoghurt.

Fresh Tomato and Lentil Soup
Serves 4.

1 tablespoon olive oil
700g ripe tomatoes cut into quarters
1 medium onion chopped finely
115g red split lentils
1.2 litres of vegetable stock
1 clove of garlic, crushed
1 red pepper
2 tablespoons tomato puree
Salt and freshly milled black pepper

To peel tomatoes, score the skin into quarters and place in a large bowl of boiling water. The skins will lift at the edges, then gently peel.

Heat the olive oil in a pan. Cook the garlic, red pepper and onion until soft. Add the tomatoes, let them cook for a few minutes then add the tomato puree, lentils and stock. Stir, cover and simmer for about 30 minutes. Season to taste, blend, reheat and serve garnished with a little chopped parsley.

Sweet Potato Soup
Serves 4

12 oz sweet potatoes, chopped into chunks
2 large leeks, topped, tailed and chopped finely
1 large onion, chopped
1 mild green chilli, de-seeded and finely chopped
1 vegetable stock cube
2 pints water

Put vegetable stock cube into a large saucepan with 2 pints of water. Add all the vegetables and chopped chilli to pan, season generously and bring to the boil with pan covered. Reduce heat and simmer for 20 – 25 minutes, with the lid half on, until all the vegetables are completely soft. Take off the heat, cool slightly and liquidise in 3 or 4 batches.

This can be served hot or cold. If the soup is too thick, add some water or milk. If serving cold, gently stir in some fromage frais or leave it floating on top with some chopped chives.

Easy, Low-fat Gazpacho
Serves 4.

2 tins of chopped tomatoes
½ chopped small cucumber
2 or 3 spring onions, peeled and chopped
½ red or green pepper, de-seeded and chopped
2 cloves of garlic, crushed
1 tablespoon of olive oil
1½ tablespoons of wine vinegar
1 heaped teaspoon of mixed herbs (fresh herbs are best, but dry will do)
black pepper to taste

Simply put everything in a liquidiser or food processor and blend until smooth. Taste, add salt and pepper and pour into a bowl. Add water (up to ½ a pint as required). Chill well before serving. You can garnish with chopped cucumber and peppers and add a couple of ice cubes if you want to.

This soup keeps well in the fridge and can be eaten as often as you want.

It is also a good way to eat vegetables as it is not cooked and contains lots of nutrients.

Light Lunches

Fresh Pasta with Salmon Sauce
Cook the pasta.
Dry pan, fry a small fillet of salmon, flake into half a cup of fromage frais.
Add squeeze of lemon juice, teaspoon ketchup or tomato puree and black pepper.
Drain pasta, add the sauce and garnish with fresh herbs.

Trout Fillet on a Bed of Spinach with Scallop Potatoes
Fry the trout in a dry pan.
Use baby salad spinach leaves – they cook/steam in 3 minutes.
Slice new potatoes, add a dash of soy sauce and black pepper.
Microwave them in cling-wrapped covered dish for approximately 4 minutes.

Wild Mushrooms on Granary Toast
Sauté the mushrooms in a little soy sauce.
Add a chopped tomato.
Top the toast and sprinkle with a little fresh, Parmesan cheese.

Pitta Bread Stuffed with Tofu and Vegetable Stir-Fry
Toast the wholemeal pitta bread lightly (they keep well in the freezer).
In a little sesame oil, dry fry 2 chopped tomatoes, half a cup of shredded leeks, a cup of finely chopped mushrooms, a tablespoon of tomato puree, a good dash of soy sauce and freshly ground black pepper.
Finally, add the tofu to the pan, with a scraping of fresh ginger.

Provençal Fish Stew served with Warm Bread
Pop the bread in a hot oven to warm.
Poach a fillet of white fish in a tin of tomatoes with a few chopped olives, a little garlic, black pepper and a handful of prawns.
Sprinkle with freshly chopped parsley.
Serve with green salad with a dash of balsamic vinegar.

Quick, Quick Risotto
Mix 6 tablespoons cooked brown rice with 50g cooked and diced chicken breast, 25g cooked peas, 50g diced green/red pepper, 50g sweetcorn and season.
Add ½ teaspoon dried mixed Italian herbs.
Re-heat in microwave.

Main Meals

Chicken Risotto with Asparagus and Mushrooms
Serves 6

5 skinless chicken breast fillets – sliced into strips
A spray of olive oil
1 stick of celery, chopped
1 large onion, sliced
1 small carrot, grated
1 bunch of asparagus
1 glass of white wine
1 clove garlic, crushed
250g button mushrooms, sliced
100g shitake mushrooms, pre-soaked and sliced
1½ tablespoons of fresh parsley, chopped
500g brown rice
1 vegetable stock cube

Cook the rice in the vegetable stock. Heat a large, deep frying pan, fry the onion, carrot, celery and garlic. Add the chicken, the wine, mushrooms, cover and simmer until tender. Steam the asparagus and cut into 3cm pieces. When the rice is cooked, add to the frying pan with the parsley and asparagus.

Chicken and Broccoli
Serves 6

150g broccoli
2 tablespoons half-fat spread
1 onion, chopped
2 courgettes, sliced
100g mushrooms, sliced
100g plain flour
Two thirds of a cup semi-skimmed milk
150ml chicken stock
300g cooked chicken, cubed

Steam broccoli. In a large saucepan melt half-fat spread over low heat. Add the onion, courgettes and mushrooms, cover and cook for 10 minutes. Stir in the flour and cook for 1 minute. Add milk and stock and slowly bring to the boil. Stir until mixture thickens. Add broccoli, chicken, salt and pepper. Simmer for 5 minutes.

Spicy Prawn Pasta
Serves 4

8 – 10 large prawns per person
1 clove garlic
½ teaspoon of red chilli sauce
2 teaspoons of soy sauce
1 cup of diced ham
½ cup of red or white wine
1 cup of cherry tomatoes chopped into quarters
1 cup of spring onions, finely chopped
4 cups of dry pasta
½ cup of fresh parsley, chopped
1 vegetable stock cube
Juice of half a lemon
Black pepper

Cook the pasta in boiling water with the stock cube until al dente.

While the pasta is cooking, marinate the prawns and ham in the soy sauce and lemon juice.

Into a pan add the wine, garlic and spring onions. Simmer for a few minutes. Turn off the heat, add the tomatoes and add the prawn mixture. Drain the pasta and serve with the sauce, garnish with the parsley. Add black pepper to taste.

Tuna and Chilli Beans
Serves 6.

150ml very low-fat fromage frais
½ cup reduced calorie mayonnaise
2 tablespoons chilli powder
2 tablespoons fresh chopped mixed herbs
3 sticks of celery, sliced
400g can of tuna in brine
400g red kidney beans
Parsley to garnish

In a bowl mix fromage frais, mayonnaise, chilli powder and herbs. Add celery, tuna, red kidney beans and mix well.

Chill until ready to serve.

Garnish with parsley and serve with freshly cooked complex carbohydrate.

Peperonata
Serves 4

6 small or 4 large peppers (assorted colours), quartered and seeded
4 tablespoons olive oil
2 onions, skinned and finely sliced
1 clove garlic, skinned and crushed
400g tomatoes, skinned, quartered and seeded
2 tablespoons vinegar (balsamic or wine vinegar is best)
Salt and pepper

Heat the oil in a large, heavy pan then stir in the onions. Cook for about 5 minutes until they are soft, then add the garlic and peppers. Cook for 15 minutes or until the peppers are soft. Stir in the tomatoes and cook for 10 minutes. Stir in the vinegar and add salt and pepper to taste. This makes a fairly dry dish. To vary it, after cooking you can add a tin of chopped tomatoes, or a carton of fresh vegetarian pasta sauce – a tomato based chilli or pepper sauce goes particularly well.

Serve with brown rice, jacket potatoes or wholemeal bread. Sprinkle cheese on top if required.

Four Seasons Pizza
Serves 4

1 pizza base (wholemeal, if not, Italian thin)
4 teaspoons sun dried tomato paste
4 teaspoons tomato puree
1 tin of chopped tomatoes, drained of juice
1 small red onion, thinly sliced
6 black olives, sliced
1 teaspoon mixed herbs
2 tablespoons fresh chopped basil
75g cooked peeled prawns
50g mushrooms, sliced
½ red pepper, thinly sliced
½ green pepper, thinly sliced
50g sweetcorn
150g grated strong cheese

Preheat oven to 200 C/400 F/Gas 6. Place the pizza base on a piece of foil on a baking tray. Spread the tomato paste, tomato puree and the drained tinned tomatoes. Sprinkle half of the cheese, then arrange the rest of the ingredients including the herbs. Scatter the remaining cheese and cook for 25 minutes until the top is bubbling and golden brown.

Pasta with Tuna and Prawns
Serves 6

450g pasta shells, wholemeal or Italian
1 vegetable stock cube
Spray olive oil
1 large red onion, finely chopped
1 red pepper, seeded and diced
1 celery stick, finely chopped
2 carrots, peeled and grated
2 tablespoons of tomato puree
2 tablespoons of honey
1 teaspoon of black pepper
2 tablespoons of anchovy paste
1 teaspoon of oregano
1 teaspoon of dried basil
1 glass of red wine
400g can chopped tomatoes
400g tinned tuna in brine
100g peeled cooked prawns
2 firm tomatoes, sliced
1 tablespoon of fresh parmesan cheese, grated finely
1 tablespoon of chopped parsley

Pre-heat the oven to 180C.

Cook the pasta in the stock until al dente. Drain and place in a large oven-proof dish. While the pasta is cooking, in a large saucepan, sauté the onion in a spray of olive oil. Add red pepper and the grated carrot. Mix together the tomato puree, honey, black pepper, anchovy paste, oregano and dried basil with the red wine, and add to the pan. Add the tin of tomatoes and simmer for 20 minutes.

Drain the tuna from the brine and flake into large chunks, add to the sauce with the prawns. Heat this gently for 3 to 4 minutes. Pour the sauce over the pasta. Top with the sliced tomatoes, parmesan cheese and parsley. Cook for 10 minutes in the oven.

Serve with green salad.

Orange and Cinnamon Pork
Serves 4

Spray of olive oil
4 lean pork chops well trimmed of all fat
1 large onion, sliced
2 cloves of garlic or 1 teaspoon of garlic paste
1 teaspoon fresh root ginger
1 yellow pepper
2 teaspoons of cinnamon
3 teaspoons of coriander
2 teaspoons of cumin
2 tablespoons of plain flour
1 glass of white wine
150ml of vegetable stock
150ml of orange juice
2 tablespoons of tomato paste
113.5g ready to eat dried apricots
2 medium oranges, sliced
Ground black pepper

Heat a large frying pan, dry fry the meat both sides to seal it, remove and place to one side. Spray the pan with olive oil, slowly fry the garlic, onion and yellow pepper until soft. Stir in the plain flour, add the spices, tomato paste, apricots and black pepper. Gradually add the stock, wine and orange juice. Bring the mixture to the boil, reduce heat, add the meat, cover and simmer gently for about 30 minutes until meat is tender.

Serve with couscous or brown rice.

Mediterranean Chicken Crepes
Serves 2.

1 cup wholemeal plain flour
1 free range egg
1½ cups of low fat milk
Olive oil cooking spray
2 teaspoons of pesto

1 small onion, finely chopped
2 courgettes, grated
1 red pepper, seeded and sliced
1 garlic clove, crushed
Small can of tomatoes
8 black olives, sliced
2 skinless chicken breasts, boiled and sliced
Fresh herbs of your choice
Salt and black pepper

Sift the flour into a mixing bowl and add a pinch of salt. Pour in some of the milk, add the egg and pesto, whisk together gradually beating in the remaining milk. Heat a large, flat frying pan, spray with oil, pour a small amount of mixture into the pan, roll around until it thinly covers most of the pan, add more mixture if necessary. Flip over when the base is light brown and cook for a few more minutes. Slide the crepe onto a plate and keep warm in the oven. Once you have cooked another one you can stack it on top of the previous crepe.

Brown the onion and garlic in a pan with a spray of olive oil. Then add the other ingredients with the courgette last. Simmer until the peppers are soft. Season to taste.

Spoon some of the ratatouille mixture into each crepe and roll.
Serve with a green salad.

Stir Fry Tofu with Sesame Seeds and Vegetables
Serves 4

285g tofu
2 garlic cloves, crushed
2 tablespoons soy sauce
Black pepper
15g sesame seeds
4 teaspoons sunflower or corn oil
175g carrots, cut into thin matchsticks
175g baby sweetcorn, halved lengthways
225g thin asparagus spears
225g yellow peppers, cut into thin strips
175g mange tout, halved crossways
175g bean sprouts
Salt
6 tablespoons sweet and sour sauce
175g Thai noodles, cooked according to packet instructions

Drain the tofu and cut it into 24 cubes. Place in a shallow bowl. Blend together the garlic, soy sauce and black pepper. Pour over the tofu pieces and toss gently. Marinate for ½ hour.

Place the sesame seeds in a hot non-stick frying pan and toast until golden brown, stirring all the time. Remove from the heat and transfer to a plate. Heat half the oil in a large non-stick wok or frying pan. Add the marinated tofu and stir-fry until lightly coloured. Remove from the pan and keep warm.

Add the remaining sunflower or corn oil and stir-fry the carrot matchsticks for 1 minute. Then add the sweetcorn, asparagus spears and pepper strips and stir fry for 2 minutes. Add the mange tout and stir fry for 1 minute.

Finally, add the bean sprouts, a little salt and the sweet and sour sauce. Stir fry them for one minute. Scatter the toasted sesame seeds over the top and serve the stir-fry with the rice noodles.

Barbecued Chicken Teriyaki
Serves 4

400g chicken thigh fillets, skinned and trimmed of fat
3 tablespoons teriyaki marinade
Black pepper and salt
400g aubergine, cut in 1 ½ cm slices
1 tablespoon sunflower oil or corn oil
2 spring onions, very thinly sliced
150g natural low fat yoghurt
225g ciabatta bread

Cut each chicken thigh into 4 pieces. Place in a large food bag. Add the marinade and pepper. Secure the top. Set aside to marinate for 3 hours. Cover all the chicken with the marinade.

1 hour before you are ready to start cooking, place the aubergine slices in a colander and sprinkle with salt. Toss well and place over a bowl to catch the juices. When ready to cook, rinse the aubergines well in cold water to remove excess salt, then pour over boiling water. Dry well on kitchen paper. Place the aubergine slices on a baking sheet and brush half the oil over the uppermost side. Thread the marinated chicken pieces on to 4 metal skewers. Brush with the marinade and place on the barbecue. Surround the chicken by the aubergine slices, oiled side down. Cook for 7 to 8 minutes. Brush the uppermost side of the aubergines with the remaining oil and the chicken pieces with the remaining marinade.

Turn over and cook for a further 8 minutes. Juices run clear when meat is cooked. Toss the thinly sliced spring onions into the yoghurt. When the aubergines are cooked, add these to the yoghurt and mix well. Serve the chicken teriyaki with the aubergines and the ciabatta bread.

Crisp Fried Chicken
Serves 4

350g chicken breast fillets, skinless
25g polenta
Salt and black pepper
450g tiny new potatoes, scrubbed and halved
700g courgettes, sliced diagonally
3 tablespoons olive oil
3 tablespoons balsamic vinegar
2 teaspoons thin honey
1 ½ tablespoons soy sauce
2 garlic cloves, crushed
4 tablespoons chopped dill or chives

Wipe the chicken breasts on kitchen paper to dry. Cut diagonally into thin strips. Set aside.

Mix polenta, salt and pepper in a bowl and stir in chicken till evenly coated. Set aside. Boil potatoes in lightly salted water. Meanwhile steam courgettes till just done. While the vegetables are cooking, prepare dressing. Blend together 1 tablespoon of oil, vinegar, honey, soy sauce and garlic in a large bowl. Add the chopped herbs to dressing. Set aside. Drain potatoes and courgettes thoroughly when cooked. Set aside but keep both warm.

Heat remaining olive oil in a large, heavy-based non-stick frying pan. When oil is very hot, toss in coated chicken pieces and fry, stirring all the time till the meat is cooked right through. This should only take a couple of minutes since the meat is thinly sliced. Turn the heat right down, cover frying pan and cook for another minute.

Remove from the pan and toss chicken and vegetables in dressing and mix thoroughly. Serve warm.

Spicy Noodle Salad With Chicken
Serves 4

500g chicken breast
1 packet Thai noodles
1 garlic clove, chopped
1 large red chilli, de-seeded and minced
half bunch coriander, well washed, drained with some stalk
½ teaspoon sugar
1 cm piece of ginger, peeled and minced
4 tablespoons soy sauce
lemon or lime juice
1 carrot, peeled and cut into very thin strips
1 spring onion, cut into very thin strips
1 tablespoon sunflower oil
1 tablespoon sesame oil

Marinate
1 tablespoon sesame oil
2 to 3 tablespoons soy sauce   } Pour over chicken
Garlic
Ginger

Cut chicken breast into small pieces (2 to 3 cm) and marinade for 15 minutes. Make dressing for salad by heating soy sauce, chilli, ginger and lemon or lime in pan and bring to boil. Leave aside to cool. Prepare rice noodles – place in pan, cover with boiling water, leave for 5 minutes. Drain well. Heat wok or pan, add sunflower oil and heat. Remove chicken from marinate and stir-fry for 3 minutes. Sprinkle coriander over the noodles. Add strips of carrots and onions. Drizzle with sesame oil.

Puddings

Pear, Apple and Cinnamon Crumble
Serves 6

400g can unsweetened pears in fruit juice
225g eating apples, peeled, cored and thinly sliced
1 to 2 teaspoons ground cinnamon
225g no-added-sugar muesli
50g sultanas
50g melted low fat spread

Pre-heat the oven to 350 F/180 C/gas mark 4.

Drain pears, reserving juice, and chop roughly. Then place in an oven-proof dish, mix together well and put aside. To make crumble mixture, mix together muesli, sultanas and melted low fat spread, spoon crumble mixture over fruit, pressing down lightly. Pour the reserved pear juice over crumble. Bake for 30 to 45 minutes or till crumble mixture is golden brown. Serve crumble hot or cold with low fat custard or low fat ice cream.

Spicy Bread Pudding
Serves 6

6 medium slices wholemeal bread
25g low fat spread
3 tablespoons no-added-sugar apricot jam
50g sultanas
50g ready to eat dried apricots, rough chopped
600ml semi-skimmed milk
2 size 3 eggs
1 rounded teaspoon ground mixed spice

Pre-heat oven to 325 F/170 C/gas mark 3.

Remove and discard crusts from bread. Spread one side of each slice with low fat spread, the other with jam. Cut each slice into fingers. Place half the bread fingers in a lightly greased oven-proof dish, mix together the sultanas and apricots and sprinkle over the bread. Top with remaining bread fingers, low fat spread side up. Whisk together milk, eggs and mixed spice and strain into the dish over bread. Leave to stand for 30 minutes to allow the bread to soak up some of the liquid. Bake for 45 to 60 minutes till set and golden brown. Serve hot or cold with fresh fruit or low fat fromage frais.

Raspberry Fluff
Serves 6

600ml unsweetened apple juice
15g packet sugar-free raspberry jelly crystals
275g raspberries
450g 8% fat natural fromage frais
Mint sprigs to garnish

Pour apple juice into a saucepan and bring to the boil, then remove from heat. Sprinkle jelly crystals over apple juice and stir till dissolved. Leave to cool. Place raspberries and fromage frais in a blender or food processor and blend till smooth. Gradually blend in the cooled jelly mixture till well combined. Pour mixture into 1 large or 6 individual serving dishes and chill till set. Garnish with mint sprigs before serving.

Quick Pudding Ideas

Poached pear in orange juice and a splash of port, decorated with a tablespoon of grated dark chocolate.

Wholewheat semolina cooked with soya milk and a few drops of almond essence. Serve with a teaspoon of sugar-free apricot jam.

Long grain brown rice pudding made with cooked brown rice, re-heated with apple juice, some raisins and a teaspoon of cinnamon.

Melon balls served with raspberry sorbet.

Jelly made with gelatine or vegetable gelling powder, freshly squeezed orange juice and grated apple.

Baked slices of fresh pineapple (10 minutes in a hot oven) sprinkled with a teaspoon of soft brown sugar.

Sorbet made from white wine.

Summer fruit salad, strawberries, grapes, melon, nectarines and bananas garnished with fresh mint.

Exotic fruit salad, fresh pineapple, kiwi fruit, grapes, mango, pawpaw and banana. In a cup pour over two teaspoons of grated ginger and two teaspoons of honey, four tablespoons of hot water and add to the fruit. Serve with yoghurt.

Warm strawberries tossed in a hot frying pan with a dash of maple syrup and a splash of white wine or sherry.

Baked apple stuffed with raisins, served with fromage frais.

Rhubarb Pie: stew rhubarb with juice and the zest of an organic orange and a little honey. Pour into an oven-proof dish, top with 2 or 3 sheets of filo pastry and bake in a hot oven for 15 minutes. Dust with icing sugar and a little nutmeg.

Lighten Up

PO Box 383
Twickenham
TW1 4EZ

Tel: 0181 744 9242
Fax: 0181 744 0553
Email: info@lightenup.co.uk

Or visit our website:
www.lightenup.co.uk

Workshops and Courses

Eight-week evening courses (two hours a week, usually on Monday nights) are running in North and South London alternately throughout the year.

One-day workshops, from 10.00am to 5.00pm, one Saturday or Sunday each month, in North or South London.

Workshops outside London

Later in 1999 and in 2000, Pete will be giving one-day workshops in various parts of the country. Call us for details.

Audio Tapes

Pete Cohen's first tape, on which he talks you through his techniques, is now available by mail order from the above address at £9.99 and £1.50 postage and packing.

TV, Radio, Magazines and Newspapers

Pete writes regularly for some magazines and appears regularly in all the media. Watch out for him!

Slimming With Pete

If you haven't seen it yet, now is the time to read the first Lighten Up book, *Slimming With Pete*. The story of Pete's first slimming group and their trials and triumphs is available from bookshops as well as by mail order at £9.99 and £2.50 postage and packing.

Let us know what you think:

We would love to hear from you. Please contact Maria or Judith by mail, phone, fax or email and let us have your feedback.

Notes

Notes

Notes

Notes

Notes

Notes

Crown House Publishing Limited
Crown Buildings,
Bancyfelin,
Carmarthen, Wales, UK, SA33 5ND.
Telephone: +44 (0) 1267 211880
Facsimile: +44 (0) 1267 211882
e-mail: bshine@crownhouse.co.uk
Website: www.crownhouse.co.uk

We trust you enjoyed this title from our range of bestselling books for professional and general readership. All our authors are professionals of many years' experience, and all are highly respected in their own field. We choose our books with care for their content and character, and for the value of their contribution of both new and updated material to their particular field. Here is a list of all our other publications.

Change Management Excellence: *Putting NLP To Work In The 21st Century*
by Martin Roberts PhD   Hardback   £25.00

Dreaming Realities: *A Spiritual System To Create Inner Alignment Through Dreams*
by John Overdurf & Julie Silverthorn   Paperback   £9.99

Ericksonian Approaches: *A Comprehensive Manual*
by Rubin Battino & Thomas L South PhD   Hardback   £25.00

Figuring Out People: *Design Engineering With Meta-Programs*
by Bob G. Bodenhamer & L. Michael Hall   Paperback   £12.99

Gold Counselling, Second Edition: *The Practical Psychology With NLP*
by Georges Philips & Lyn Buncher   Paperback   £16.99

Grieve No More, Beloved: *The Book Of Delight*
by Ormond McGill   Hardback   £9.99

Hypnotherapy Training In The UK: *An Investigation Into The Development Of Clinical Hypnosis Training Post-1971*
by Shaun Brookhouse   Spiralbound   £9.99

Influencing With Integrity: *Management Skills For Communication & Negotiation*
by Genie Z Laborde   Paperback   £12.50

Instant Relaxation: *How To Reduce Stress At Work, At Home And In Your Daily Life*
by L. Michael Hall with Debra Lederer   Paperback   £8.99

The Magic Of Mind Power: *Awareness Techniques For The Creative Mind*
by Duncan McColl   Paperback   £8.99

A Multiple Intelligences Road To An ELT Classroom
by Michael Berman   Paperback   £19.99

Multiple Intelligences Poster Set
by Jenny Maddern   Nine posters   £19.99

The New Encyclopedia Of Stage Hypnotism
by Ormond McGill   Hardback   £29.99

Now It's YOUR Turn For Success! *Training And Motivational Techniques For Direct Sales*
And Multi-Level Marketing
by Richard Houghton and Janet Kelly   Paperback   £9.99

Peace Of Mind Is A Piece Of Cake
by Michael Mallows & Joseph Sinclair   Paperback   £8.99

The POWER Process: *An NLP Approach To Writing*
by Sid Jacobson & Dixie Elise Hickman   Paperback   £12.99

Precision Therapy: *A Professional Manual Of Fast And Effective Hypnoanalysis Techniques*
by Duncan McColl PhD   Paperback   £15.00

Rapid Cognitive Therapy: *The Professional Therapists' Guide To Rapid Change Work*
by Georges Philips & Terrence Watts   Paperback   £20.00

Scripts & Strategies In Hypnotherapy
by Roger P. Allen   Hardback   £19.99

The Secrets Of Magic: *Communicational Excellence For The 21st Century*
by L. Michael Hall   Paperback   £14.99

Seeing The Unseen: *A Past Life Revealed Through Hypnotic Regression*
by Ormond McGill   Paperback   £12.99

Slimming With Pete: *Taking The Weight Off Body AND Mind*
by Pete Cohen & Judith Verity   Paperback   £9.99

Smoke-Free And No Buts!
by Geoff Ibbotson & Ann Williamson   Paperback   £5.99

Solution States: *A Course In Solving Problems In Business With The Power Of NLP*
by Sid Jacobson   Paperback   £12.99

The Sourcebook Of Magic: *A Comprehensive Guide To NLP Techniques*
by L. Michael Hall & Barbara Belnap   Paperback   £14.99

The Spirit Of NLP: *The Process, Meaning And Criteria For Mastering NLP*
by L. Michael Hall   Paperback   £12.99

Sporting Excellence: *Optimising Sports Performance Using NLP*
by Ted Garatt   Paperback   £9.99

Time-Lining: *Patterns For Adventuring In "Time"*
by Bob G. Bodenhamer & L. Michael Hall   Paperback   £14.99

The User's Manual For The Brain: *The Complete Manual For Neuro-Linguistic Programming*
   Practitioner Certification
by Bob G. Bodenhamer & L. Michael Hall   A4 binder   £30.00

Vibrations For Health And Happiness: *Everyone's Easy Guide To Stress-free Living*
by Tom Bolton   Paperback   £9.99

Order form

✱✱✱✱✱✱✱Special offer: 4 for the price of 3!✱✱✱✱✱✱✱

Buy 3 books & we'll give you a 4th title – FREE!
(free title will be book of lowest value)

Qty	Title	Qty	Title
—	Change Management Excellence	—	The POWER Process
—	Doing It With Pete	—	Precision Therapy
—	Dreaming Realities	—	Rapid Cognitive Therapy
—	Ericksonian Approaches	—	Scripts & Strategies In Hypnotherapy
—	Figuring Out People	—	The Secrets Of Magic
—	Gold Counselling Second Edition	—	Seeing The Unseen
—	Grieve No More, Beloved	—	Slimming With Pete
—	Hypnotherapy Training In The UK	—	Smoke-Free And No Buts!
—	Influencing With Integrity	—	Solution States
—	Instant Relaxation	—	The Sourcebook Of Magic
—	The Magic Of Mind Power	—	The Spirit Of NLP
—	A Multiple Intelligences Road To An ELT Classroom	—	Sporting Excellence
—	Multiple Intelligences Poster Set	—	Time-Lining
—	New Encyclopedia Of Stage Hypnotism	—	The User's Manual For The Brain
—	Now It's YOUR Turn For Success!	—	Vibrations For Health And Happiness
—	Peace Of Mind Is A Piece Of Cake		

Postage and packing

UK:	£2.50 for one book
	£4.50 for two or more books
Europe:	£3.50 per book
Rest of the world	£4.50 per book

My details:

Name: Mr/Mrs/Ms/Other (please specify)..

Address:...

....

....

Postcode: .Daytime tel:

I wish to pay by:

☐ Amex.........................☐ Visa.........................☐ Mastercard.........................☐ Switch – Issue no./Start date:.......................................

Card number: Expiry date ....

Name on card:..Signature:...

☐ cheque/postal order payable to **AA Books**

Please send me the following catalogues:

☐	Accelerated Learning (Teaching Resources)	☐	Psychotherapy/Counselling
☐	Accelerated Learning (Personal Growth)	☐	Employment Development
☐	Neuro-Linguistic Programming	☐	Business
☐	NLP Video Library – hire (UK only)	☐	Freud
☐	NLP Video Library – sales	☐	Jung
☐	Ericksonian Hypnotherapy	☐	Transactional Analysis
☐	Classical Hypnosis	☐	Parenting
☐	Gestalt Therapy	☐	Special Needs

Please fax/send to:
The Anglo American Book Company,
FREEPOST SS1340
Crown Buildings, Bancyfelin,
Carmarthen, West Wales,
United Kingdom, SA33 4ZZ,
Tel: +44 (0) 1267 211880/211886 Fax: +44 (0) 1267 211882
or e-mail your order to:
books@anglo-american.co.uk